Aravind's Atlas of
Fungal Corneal Ulcers
Clinical Features and Laboratory Identification Methods

Aravind's Atlas of
Fungal Corneal Ulcers
Clinical Features and Laboratory Identification Methods

Lalitha Prajna MD

Vijayakumar MSc

Department of Ocular Microbiology
Aravind Eye Hospital, Madurai, Tamil Nadu
India

N Venkatesh Prajna DNB, FRC (Ophth)

M Srinivasan MS

Department of Cornea and External Diseases
Aravind Eye Hospital, Madurai, Tamil Nadu
India

JAYPEE BROTHERS MEDICAL PUBLISHERS (P) LTD

New Delhi • Ahmedabad • Bengaluru • Chennai • Hyderabad • Kochi
Kolkata • Lucknow • Mumbai • Nagpur

Published by

Jitendar P Vij
Jaypee Brothers Medical Publishers (P) Ltd
B-3 EMCA House, 23/23B Ansari Road, Daryaganj
New Delhi 110 002, India
Phones: +91-11-23272143, +91-11-23272703, +91-11-23282021, +91-11-23245672
Rel: +91-11-32558559 Fax: +91-11-23276490, +91-11-23245683 e-mail: jaypee@jaypeebrothers.com
Visit our website: www.jaypeebrothers.com

Branches

- 2/B, Akruti Society, Jodhpur Gam Road Satellite
  Ahmedabad 380 015 Phones: +91-79-26926233, Rel: +91-79-32988717
  Fax: +91-79-26927094, e-mail: ahmedabad@jaypeebrothers.com
- 202 Batavia Chambers, 8 Kumara Krupa Road, Kumara Park East
  Bengaluru 560 001 Phones: +91-80-22285971, +91-80-22382956, +91-80-22372664 Rel: +91-80-32714073
  Fax: +91-80-22281761, e-mail: bangalore@jaypeebrothers.com
- 282 IIIrd Floor, Khaleel Shirazi Estate, Fountain Plaza, Pantheon Road
  Chennai 600 008 Phones: +91-44-28193265, +91-44-28194897, Rel: +91-44-32972089
  Fax: +91-44-28193231, e-mail: chennai@jaypeebrothers.com
- 4-2-1067/1-3, 1st Floor, Balaji Building, Ramkote Cross Road
  Hyderabad 500 095 Phones: +91-40-66610020, +91-40-24758498, Rel:+91-40-32940929
  Fax:+91-40-24758499, e-mail: hyderabad@jaypeebrothers.com
- No. 41/3098, B & B1, Kuruvi Building, St. Vincent Road
  Kochi 682 018, Kerala Phones: +91-484-4036109, +91-484-2395739, +91-484-2395740
  e-mail: kochi@jaypeebrothers.com
- 1-A Indian Mirror Street, Wellington Square
  Kolkata 700 013 Phones: +91-33-22651926, +91-33-22276404, +91-33-22276415,
  Rel: +91-33-32901926 Fax: +91-33-22656075, e-mail: kolkata@jaypeebrothers.com
- Lekhraj Market III, B-2, Sector-4, Faizabad Road, Indira Nagar
  Lucknow 226 016 Phones: +91-522-3040553, +91-522-3040554
  e-mail: lucknow@jaypeebrothers.com
- 106 Amit Industrial Estate, 61 Dr SS Rao Road Near MGM Hospital, Parel
  Mumbai 400 012 Phones: +91-22-24124863, +91-22-24104532
  Rel: +91-22-32926896 Fax: +91-22-24160828, e-mail: mumbai@jaypeebrothers.com
- "KAMALPUSHPA" 38, Reshimbag Opp. Mohota Science College, Umred Road
  Nagpur 440 009 (MS) Phone: Rel: +91-712-3245220 Fax: +91-712-2704275
  e-mail: nagpur@jaypeebrothers.com

Aravind's Atlas of Fungal Corneal Ulcers—Clinical Features and Laboratory Identification Methods

First Edition: **2008**

ISBN 978-81-8448-365-9

Typeset at JPBMP typesetting unit
Printed at Ajanta Offset & Packagings Ltd., New Delhi

Foreword

The World Health Organization has recognized the diseases of the cornea as one of the major causes of vision loss and blindness; next to cataract blindness. It is estimated that ocular trauma and corneal ulceration result in 1.5 to 2 million new cases of corneal blindness every year. Among the corneal diseases, fungus keratitis forms major binding eye diseases in Asia particularly in Southern parts of India. It is a very serious and painful corneal lesion which accounts for 44% of all central corneal ulcers in South India.

Early recognition of the fungal lesions of the eye will aid in appropriate treatment of the condition. More than the sophisticated technology, it is acquiring the basic information and knowledge on diagnosis and identification of the organism is the deciding factor for the proper management and prevention of corneal blindness. The clinical appearance of fungal corneal ulcers varies greatly depending on the type of organism, the duration of the disease and the severity of infection. Diagnosis of these patients is based on the clinical findings along with isolation of fungi from the ulcer site. Corneal scrapings are obtained with the specific and simple technique, staining with the available staining methods and culture in all cases of suspected fungal lesions are necessary to diagnose the lesions early and institute the appropriate treatment. During recent times very sophisticated techniques like PCR have come to the help of microbiologists for accurate diagnosis of the fungal keratitis so that the specific treatment can be given.

Ocular microbiology has developed very rapidly. This atlas has been prepared in great detail and it contains excellent colour photographs with descriptive text. Much emphasize has been laid on the methods of sample collection and various staining methods to isolate the fungal organism and technique of growing the fungi in various culture media. The clinical presentations of different types of fungal corneal lesions at various stages are clearly brought out so that the readers will have little difficulty in identification of pathology in practice.

I am very happy to observe that the authors have tried their best to describe the various types of fungal corneal ulcers with illustrative quality pictures. It is a comprehensive overview of all the aspects of fungal keratitis including the clinical presentation, diagnosis and laboratory techniques. The extensive review of the morphology and culture techniques of various fungal organisms are given vividly so that the postgraduates in ophthalmology and microbiologists will have an up-to-date knowledge on ocular fungal infection and available treatment modalities. I am sure that this Atlas with the collection of excellent photographs will help the teachers and the students as a guide for diagnosis and management of fungal corneal ulcers.

P Namperumalsamy
Chairman
Aravind Eye Care System
Madurai, Tamil Nadu, India

Preface

Fungal corneal ulcers are an important cause of ocular morbidity throughout the world. The recent epidemic in the Western world has ensured that it is now recognized universally to be a public health problem. The importance of microbiological techniques to confirm the diagnosis and thereby to plan for a appropriate therapy cannot be underestimated. In this atlas, we present the clinical features and the descriptive microbiological details of the fungi isolated from different corneal ulcers. This atlas is intended to serve as a practical guide for Ophthalmologist and Microbiologist, when confronted with clinical cases of fungal corneal ulcers.

Lalitha Prajna
Vijayakumar
N Venkatesh Prajna
M Srinivasan

Acknowledgements

- Dr Sean Socrates D'Silva for assisting in compilation of the clinical photographs.
- Dr Revathi Rajaram, Aravind Eye Hospital, Coimbatore for contribution of clinical photographs.
- Dr Sourabh Mittal, Aravind Eye Hospital, Thirunelveli for contribution of clinical photographs.
- Mr Manikandan, Ocular Microbiologist, Aravind Eye Hospital, Coimbatore for contribution of fungal photographs.
- M Rajkumar and R Jeyakrishnan for photographic expertise.
- Staff of the Department of Ocular Microbiology and Staff of the Department of Cornea and External Diseases.

Contents

CHAPTER 1

Introduction

According to the World Health Organization, corneal diseases are a major cause of vision loss and blindness, second only to cataract in overall importance. It is estimated that ocular trauma and corneal ulceration result in 1.5 to 2 million new cases of corneal blindness annually. This is a major public health problem in developing countries and infections constitute the most predominant cause. There is wide geographical variation in the epidemiological pattern of corneal ulcers across and even within countries.

A study conducted by Srinivasan et al (2004) at our institute, reported fungal keratitis as an enormous public health problem in south India. Fungi, especially Fusarium (47%) and Aspergillus (16%), were identified as the etiological agents responsible for 44% of all corneal ulcers in that study. This high prevalence of fungal pathogens in South India is significantly greater than that found in similar studies in Nepal (17%), Bangladesh (36%), Ghana (37.6%), and south Florida (35%) (Liesegang TJ et al, 1980, Upadhyay MP et al, 1991, Dunlop AA et al, 1994, Hagan M et al,1995 and Leck AK et al, 2002). In China, the incidence of fungal keratitis has increased during the past decade (Dongx, et al 1994). In temperate climates, such as Britain and the northern United States, the incidence of fungal keratitis remains very low (Coster DJ et al, 1981).

Local predisposing factors include trauma, contact lenses, and topical steroids. Other disorders, including corneal surface disorders, dry eye, bullous keratopathy, and exposure keratitis, are associated with the development of suppurative keratitis. (Tuli SS et al, 2002 and Periman LM et al., 2003). Recently, several case reports of fungal keratitis after photorefractive keratectomy and Lasik have been published (Chang CW et al, 2002, Tanure MA et al, 2000). As for systemic factors, the incidence of fungal keratitis is not particularly high in immunocompromised patients and those with diabetes (Asbell P et al,1982, Panda A et al, 1997). The importance of trauma that is often too trivial and frequently associated with plant material has been well documented in the initiation of fungal infection caused by filamentous fungi. Agricultural workers in a rural setting and people working in warehouses storing agricultural products, especially onions and groundnuts are specially at risk since the filamentous fungi are found in abundance in relation to these products.

Certain investigators have highlighted the association between the prevailing climatic conditions and the incidence of fungal keratitis. In Florida, the incidence of fungal keratitis is reportedly highest between November and March when the climate is cold, dry and windy. In India the incidence is highest in the harvesting seasons of September and October. There is less seasonal variation with regard to yeast infections.

Filamentous fungi form the major etiologic agents of fungal keratitis. *Fusarium* species (37-62%) and *Aspergillus* species (24-30%) have been implicated as main pathogens. Dematiaceous fungi have been reported to be the cause of 8 to 16.7% of cases of fungal keratitis (Hagan M et al, 1995, Bharathi MJ et al, 2003, Whitcher JP et al, 1994). The etiological agent for fungal keratitis may vary within countries—*Fusarium* species is more commonly associated with fungal keratitis in southern India, while *Aspergillus* species is more often implicated in northern India and adjoining Nepal. Most filamentous fungi associated with corneal ulceration in the tropics are found widely within the environment. Chang et al from Taiwan have reported that *Fusarium* species are common plant pathogens, particularly in corn crops or onion fields (Chang CW et al, 2002) Yeast can also cause keratitis. In a series of 24 patients from Wills Eye Hospital, Philadelphia, Candida was identified in 45.8% of cases of fungal keratitis; this probably represents the only study reporting Candida as the commonest etiologic agent of fungal keratitis (Tanure MA et al, 2000). Gopinathan et al from India have reported Candida as a rare fungal corneal pathogen (0.7%) (Gopinathan U et al, 2002). Unlike the experience of bacterial keratitis, for the past two decades the spectrum of fungal pathogens causing fungal keratitis has not changed significantly (Srinivasan M et al, 1997 and Bharathi MJ, et al, 2003).

Even though certain clinical features are pathognomonic, laboratory diagnosis is essential to confirm the findings. Laboratory diagnosis can be made by means of smear, staining and fungal culture. Although polymerase chain reaction (PCR) and confocal microscopy are being used as new rapid diagnostic methods they are expensive and not available in areas where fungal keratitis is highly prevalent (Florakis GJ et al, 1997 and Gaudio PA et al, 2002).

While means to identify etiological agents are available, the lack of effective antifungal agents often translates to an inability to treat the keratitis despite diagnosis (O'Day DM 1987, Dursun D et al, 2003, Lalitha P et al, 2006). Antifungal drug sensitivity tests need to be developed and standardized to select appropriate antifungal agents depending on the organism isolated. Until recently, only a single drug was available for the management of fungal keratitis in developing countries despite the known potential for vision impairment and blindness associated with fungal keratitis. Although emerging antifungal agents show promise, therapeutic gaps will probably persist, and further development is necessary. Priorities should be given to develop and undertake drug trials against filamentous fungal keratitis. Basic research about the role of cytokines in corneal inflammation and tissue destruction should be encouraged.

The increased incidence of fungal keratitis, coupled with a decreased availability of donor corneas in developing countries, warrants further study of the risk factors, host pathogen interactions, antifungal susceptibility testing, and newer pharmacological trials in an effort to strengthen our armamentarium to combat this potentially blinding disease.

CHAPTER

2

Clinical Presentation of Fungal Keratitis

The early lesions of fungal keratitis are quite characteristic. The symptoms are less than what the size would warrant. The symptoms are also less than that of bacterial keratitis of similar size. Some of the characteristic clinical manifestations include, dry raised surface, feathery margins, satellite lesions and posterior corneal abscess. Of these, feathery margins are very typical of fungal corneal ulcers (Figs 2.1 to 2.21).

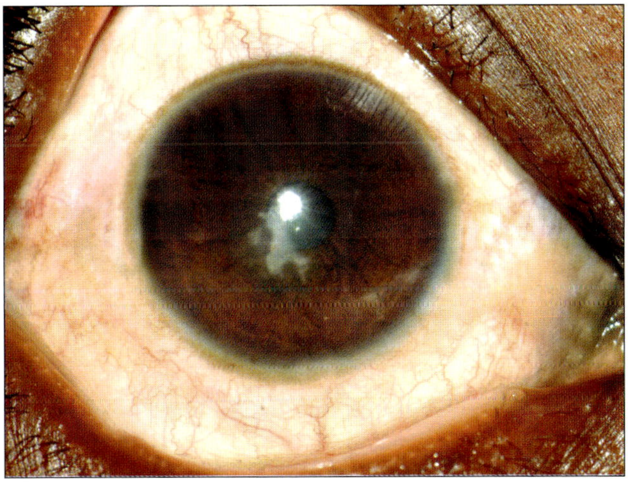

Fig. 2.1: An early fungal ulcer presenting with very mild congestion and few symptoms. In fungal keratitis the signs are disproportionately higher than the symptoms

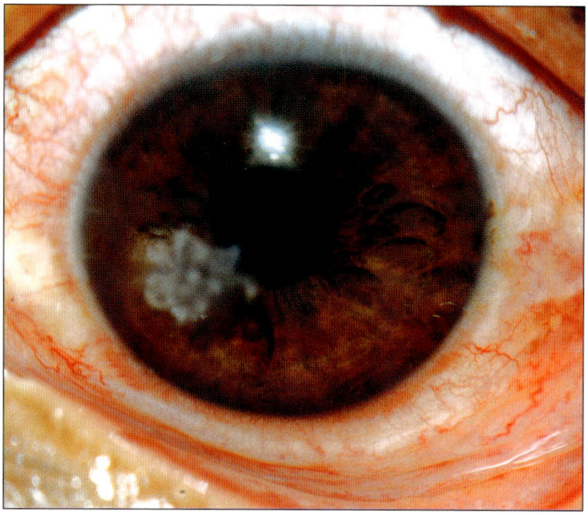

Fig. 2.2: Slit lamp photograph of fungal corneal ulcer in the early stages of the infection in which the ulcer is just beginning to progress with the typical feathery margins at the 7'O clock position. The feathery margin is pathognomonic of a fungal corneal ulcer

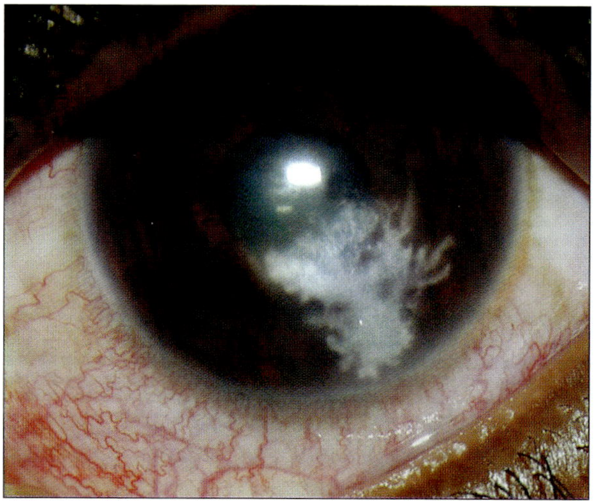

Fig. 2.3: Corneal ulcer, culture positive for *Fusarium*, in which the typical broad feathery infiltrate in the anterior stroma are progressing to become broader

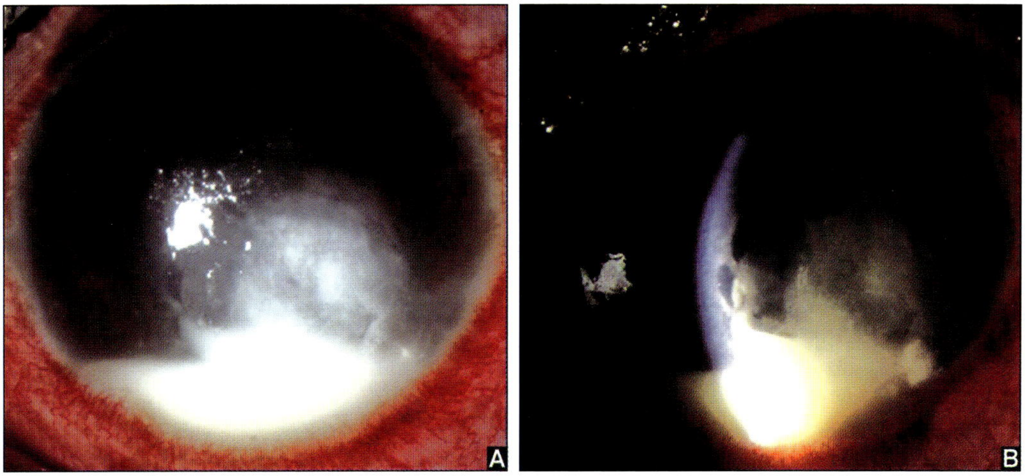

Figs 2.4A and B: *Fusarium* keratitis with endothelial exudates (white fluffy mass in the middle) forming the appearance of a double layered hypopyon

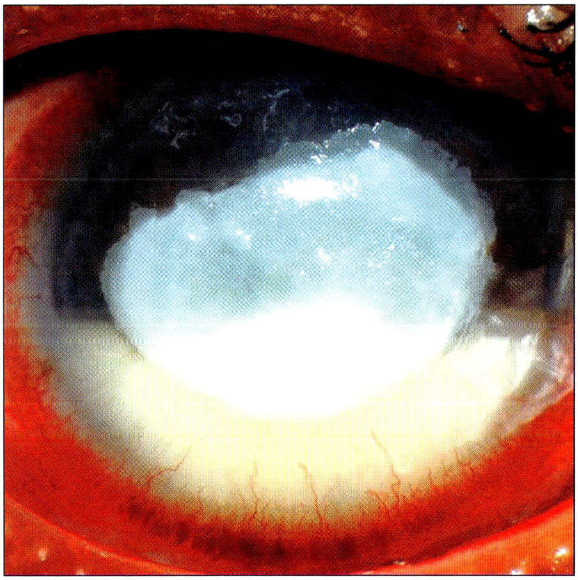

Fig. 2.5: A culture positive *Fusarium* keratitis presenting with a central thick plaque with a large hypopyon in the anterior chamber

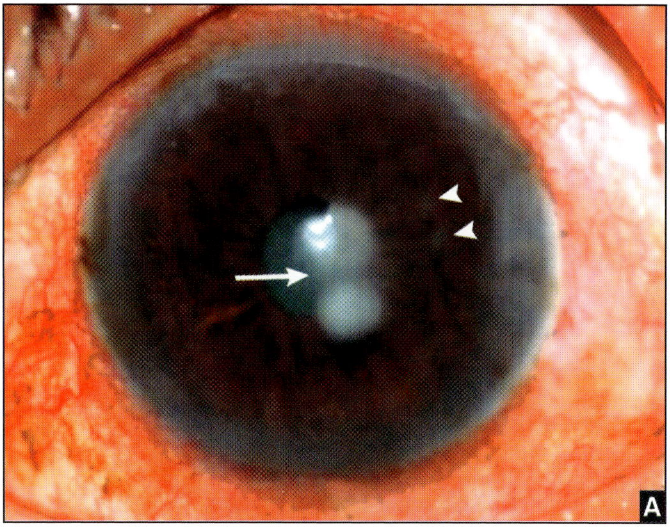

Fig. 2.6A: 10 days old fungal corneal ulcer showing two central (→) and two peripheral satellite (∢) lesions

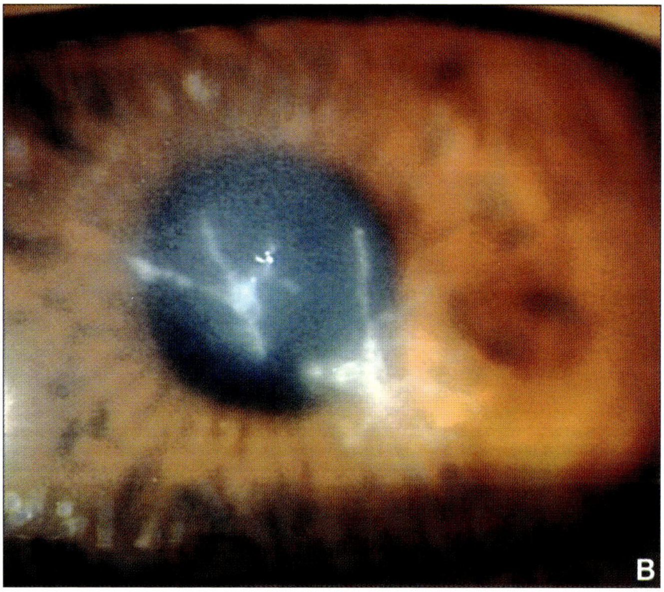

Fig. 2.6B: 10 days old clinical presentation of two feathery edged corneal lesions separated by a clear corneal region. This is an unusual presentation of a satellite lesion, which is usually round in shape

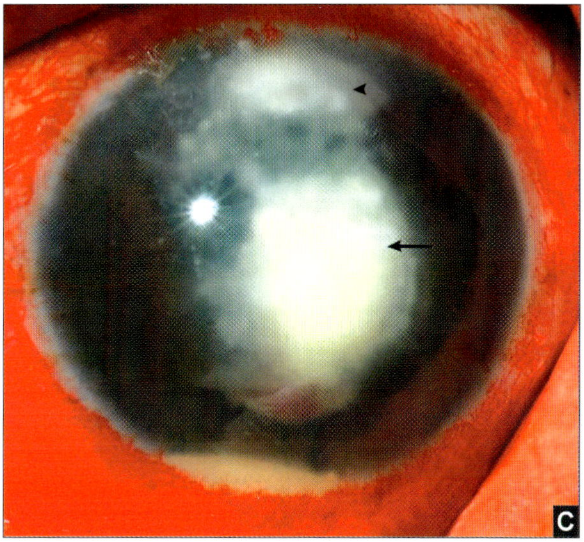

Fig. 2.6C: Satellite lesion which are pathognomic for fungal corneal ulcers (∢ Satellite lesion ← Main lesion)

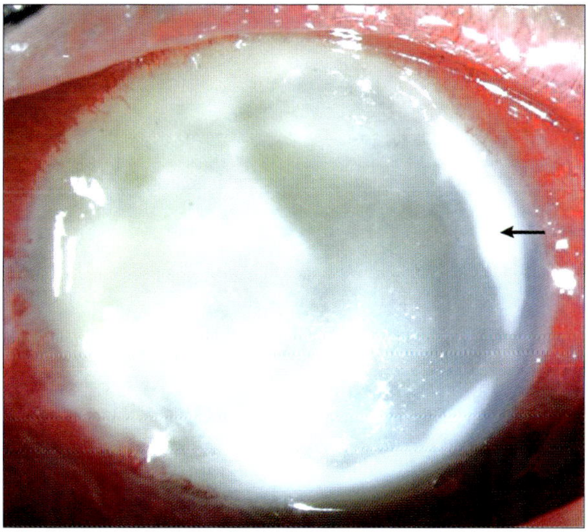

Fig. 2.7: An unusual fungal corneal ulcer that is extending up to the limbus and spreading peripherally towards the temporal aspect. The anterior chamber is filled with exudates (→ Peripherally spreading fungal ulcer)

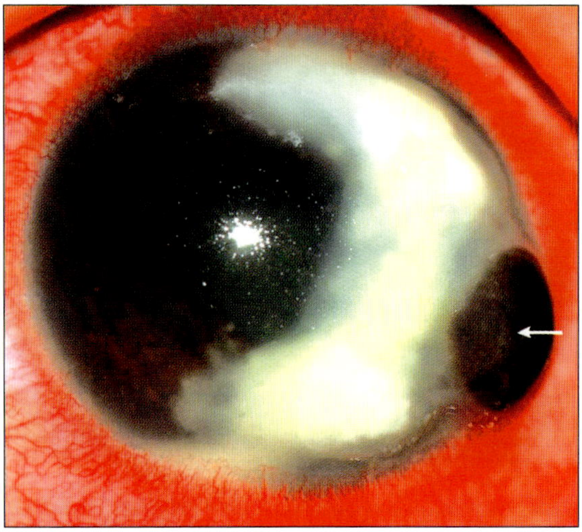

Fig. 2.8: Iris prolapse in peripheral fungal ulcer

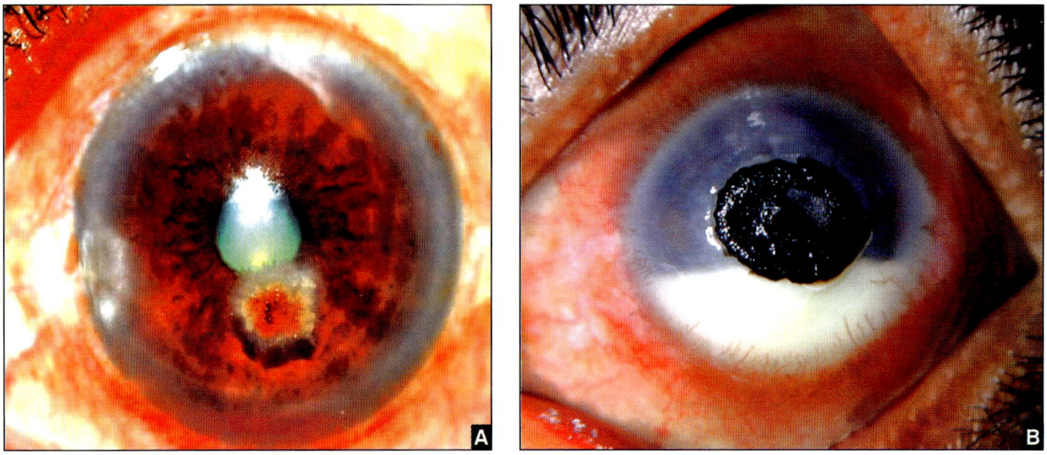

Figs 2.9A and B: These pictures show an ulcer that is brown (A) black (B) in color and caused by dematiaceous fungi that produce similar pigmentation in culture. Often the clinical presentation might be mistaken for a foreign body in the cornea due to the color and appearance

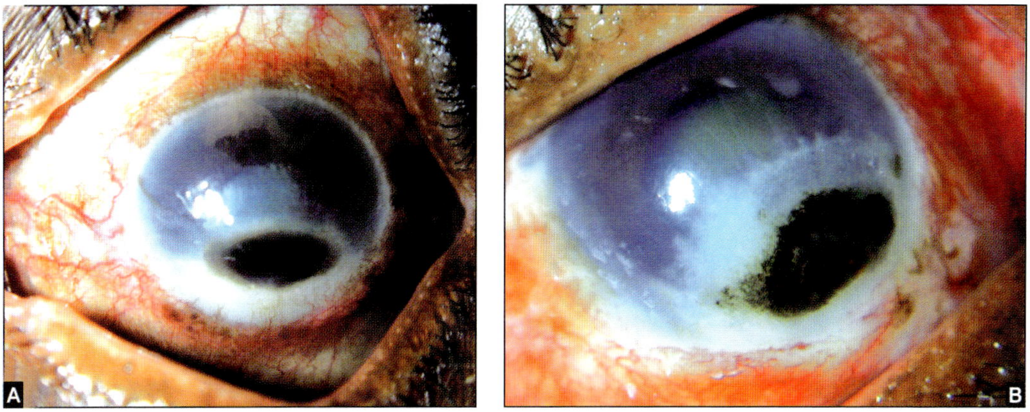

Figs 2.10A and B: This picture shows a black mass at the inferior edge that might be mistaken for iris prolapse through a perforated cornea. Examination of this lesion demonstrated this to be a fungal mass caused by dematiaceous fungi

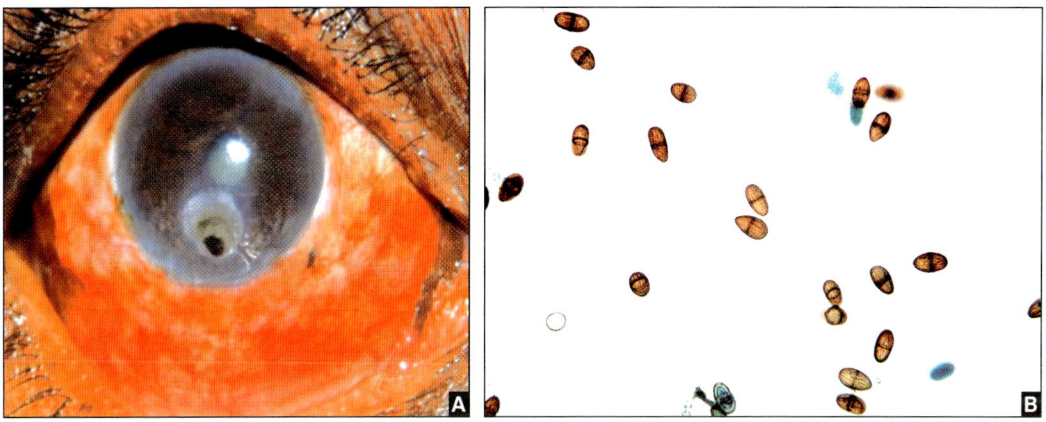

Figs 2.11A and B: This pigmented ulcer was caused by the dematiaceous fungi *Lasiodiplodia theobromae* an uncommon ocular pathogen. A. Clinical picture, B. Spores of *Lasiodiplodia theobromae*

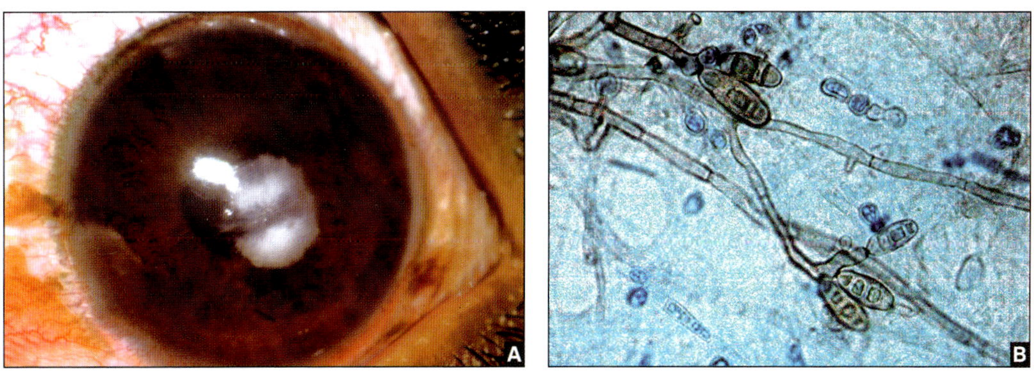

Figs 2.12A and B: Fungal corneal ulcer caused by the dematiaceous fungi *Bipolaris*, in which a white fluffy infiltrate in the stroma can be seen and the surrounding cornea is clear. A. Clinical picture, B. Spores of *Bipolaris* species

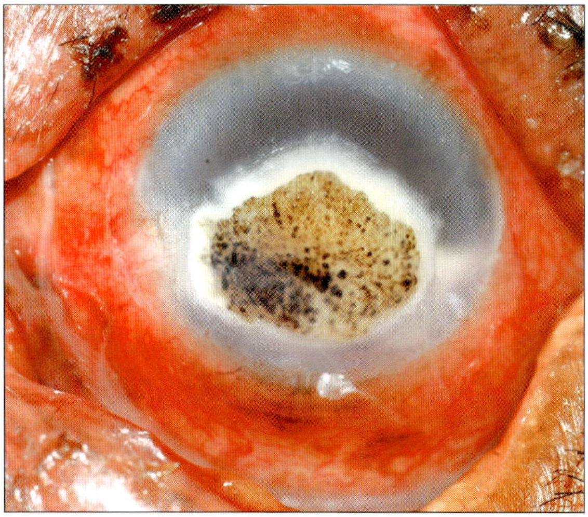

Fig. 2.13: Fungal corneal ulcer caused by the dematiaceous fungi and the pigmentation appear as leopard like brown spots on the ulcer

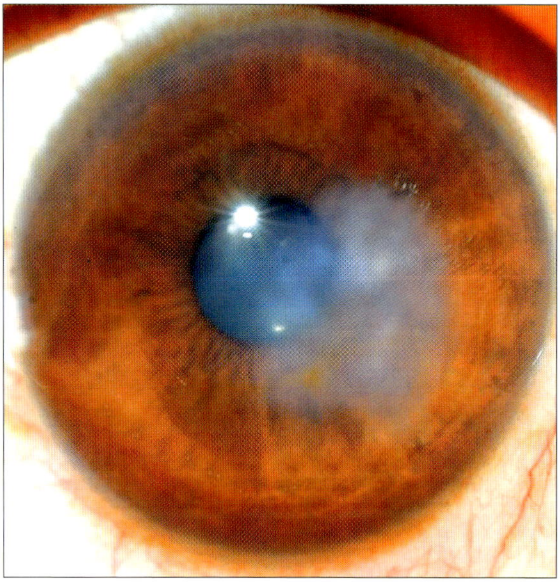

Fig. 2.14: A clinical presentation of a fungal keratitis with a disproportionately high stromal inflammation. This presentation can mimic a viral keratitis

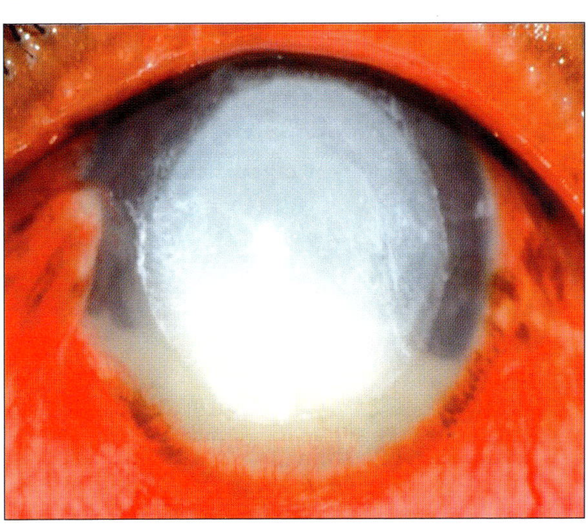

Fig. 2.15: Fungal corneal ulcer that is involving nearly the entire cornea. These types of presentations are often seen in real life situations. Etiology of the ulcers presenting at this stage cannot be diagnosed by clinical means and often require microbiological investigations to confirm the diagnosis

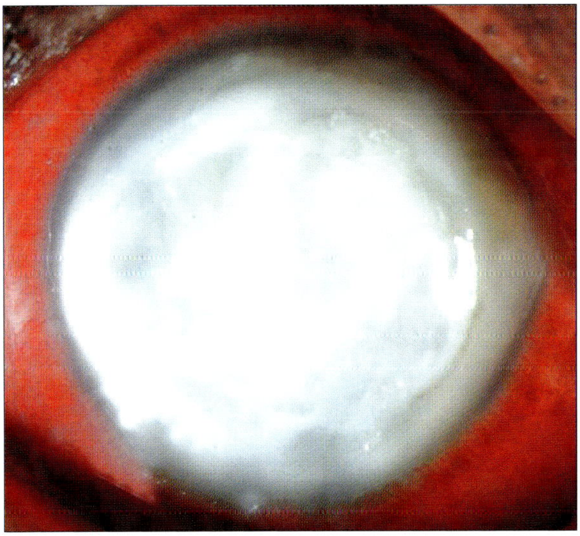

Fig. 2.16: Fungal corneal ulcers that has involved the entire cornea. The prognosis is poor and would require a penetrating keratoplasty

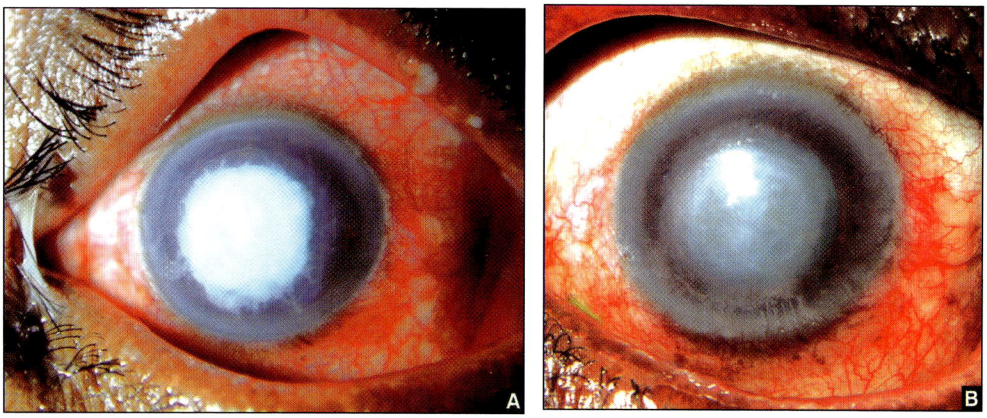

Figs 2.17A and B: A. Fungal ulcer with active infiltrate. B. Same ulcer showing signs of healing after topical natamycin therapy

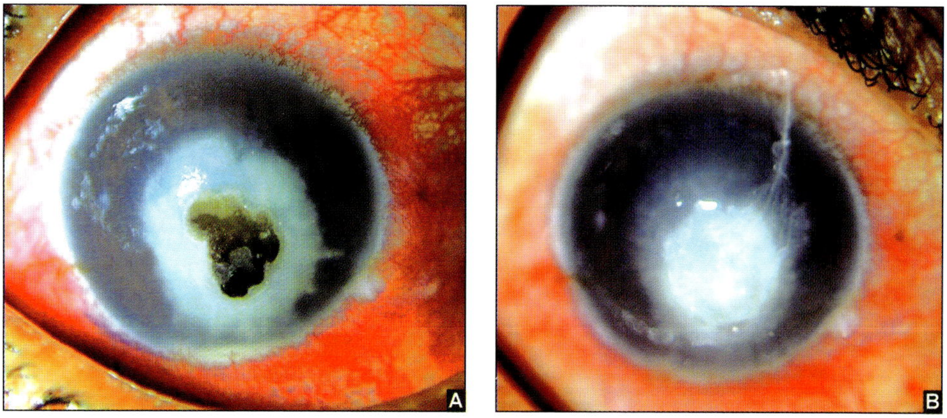

Figs 2.18A and B: A. Fungal corneal ulcer due to dematiaceous fungi, with a black mass in the center. B. Superficial keratectomy helps to debulk the fungal mass and also allows better penetration of the drug into the cornea

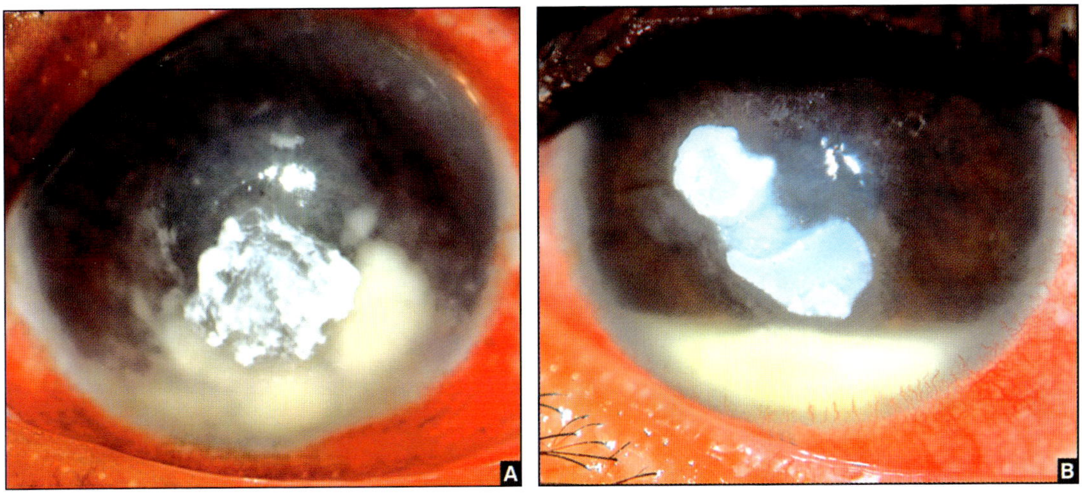

Figs 2.19A and B: Natamycin (eye drops) deposits (white plaque like structure in the center) on the cornea in a case of fungal keratitis

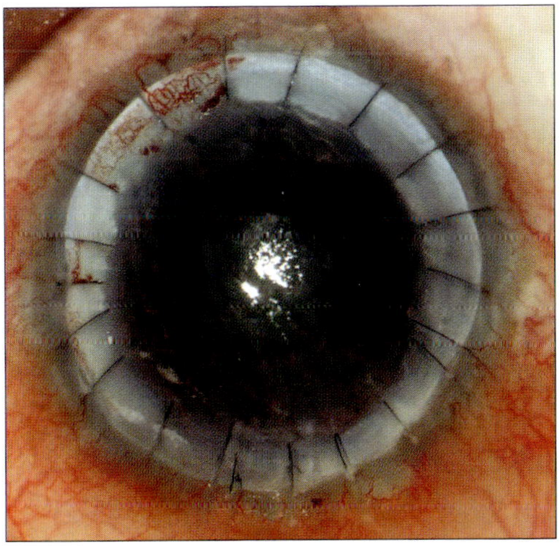

Fig. 2.20: Therapeutic keratoplasty done in a case of fungal keratitis

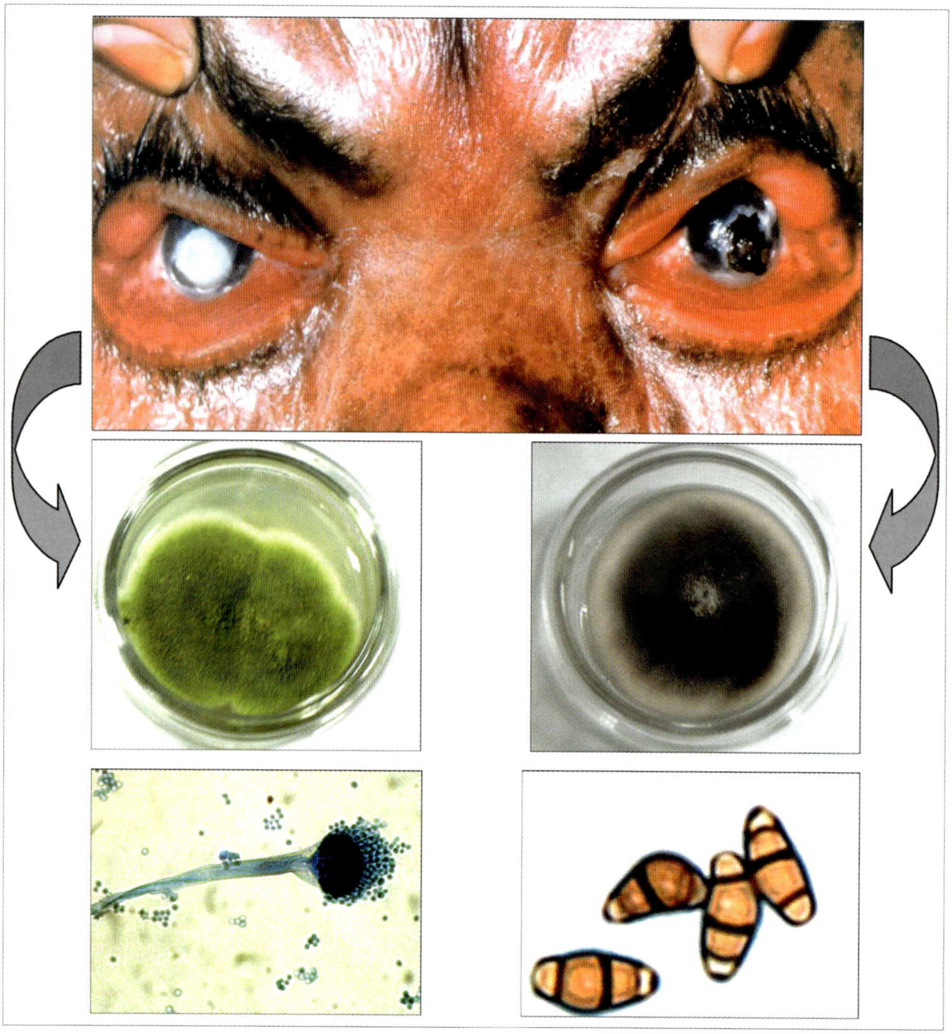

Fig. 2.21: Simultaneous bilateral fungal keratitis caused by different fungi. An interesting case report This was a 60-year-old female patient with lamellar ichthyoses who presented with simultaneous bilateral fungal keratitis caused by different fungi (One pigmented and the other non-pigmented) fungi. The interesting feature was that one eye was affected by *Aspergillus* and the fellow eye was affected by *Curvularia*. Although *Aspergillus* and *Curvularia* have been reported as causes of fungal keratitis, the simultaneous occurrence in the same patient is a curiosity. The patient was treated with topical natamycin 5 % suspension applied hourly in both eyes for five days and then two hourly. Both ulcers showed signs of healing after 10 days

(Courtesy—Prajna N Venkatesh et al, Simultaneous bilateral fungal keratitis caused by different fungi. Indian J Ophthalmol 2002;50:213-214.)

CHAPTER 3

Specimen Collection

Standard procedures followed for ocular specimen collection, culture isolation and identification of the organisms are described below.

SPECIMEN COLLECTION KIT TO BE KEPT IN THE OPHTHALMOLOGIST OFFICE

The following are the items that must be available for collecting the corneal specimens.

- Culture plates (blood agar, potato dextrose agar)
- Sterile Kimura's spatula or scraper
- Topical anesthetic agents
- Bunsen burner
- Clean glass slides
- Clean cover slips.

Corneal Scraping

Corneal scraping is performed under aseptic conditions by an ophthalmologist using a sterile Kimura spatula. The procedure is performed under magnification of a slit lamp or binocular loupe following instillation of topical anesthetic agents such as 0.5% proparacaine or 4% lignocaine.

Material obtained from scraping the leading edge and the base of each ulcer specimen are inoculated directly onto sheep blood agar, potato dextrose agar (PDA) and Brain Heart Infusion broth (BHI) without gentamycin sulphate. The material from the corneal scraping is also smeared and labeled onto slides in a thin, even manner to prepare a 10% KOH wet mount and Gram staining. In cases of suspected actinomycetes keratitis Kinyoun's method of acid fast staining is performed (Fig. 3.1). Corneal scrapings collected by an opthalmologist by using an ophthalmic microscope in shown in Figures 3.4A to F.

In some of the patients, the ulcer may be predominately in the deeper stromal lesion, with inflammatory outpourings in the anterior chamber. In such a case, a paracentesis is made using a 26 gauge needle mounted on a 2cc plastic disposable tuberculin syringe (Figs 3.2A and B).

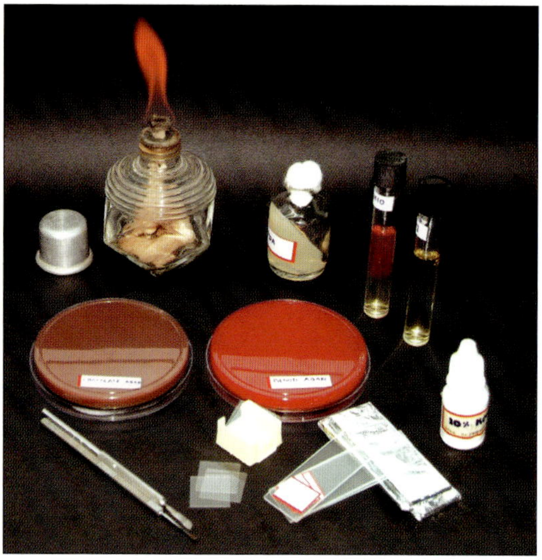

Fig. 3.1: Materials used for collecting specimens from corneal ulcers

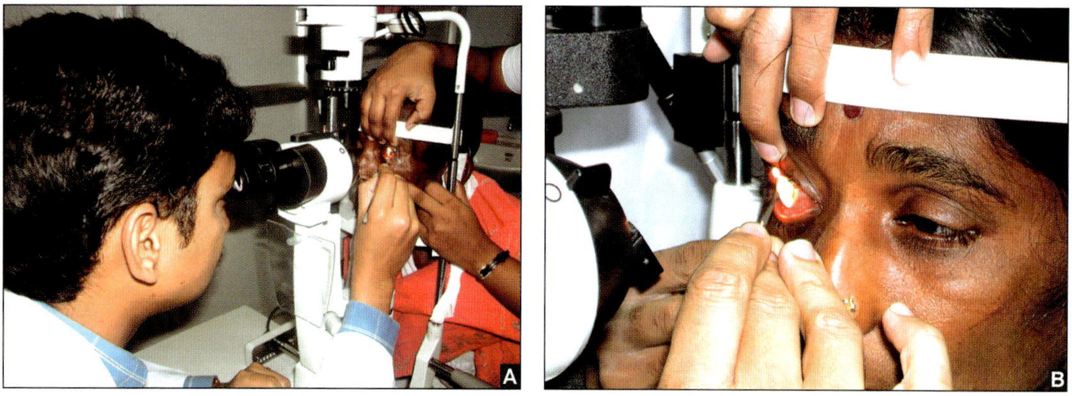

Figs 3.2A and B: Corneal scraping collected by an ophthalmologist by using slit lamp microscope

Biopsy

Deep stromal lesions and lesion with initially negative culture that may continue to progress clinically may require corneal biopsy. A corneal biopsy in the operation theater. A 3 to 5 mm circular trephine set to a depth of 0.2 to 0.3 mm can be used to outline the are to be biopsied. The edge of the specimen is lifted with a forceps and discussed. The tissue can be bisected and send for both histological analysis and culture. The base of the specimen can also be scrapped for routine culture (Fig 3.3).

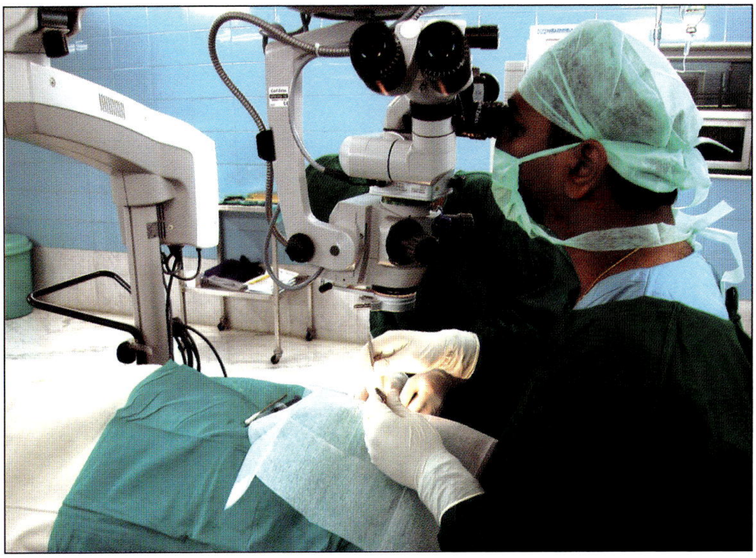

Fig. 3.3 : Corneal biopsy collected by ophthalmologist in an operation theater

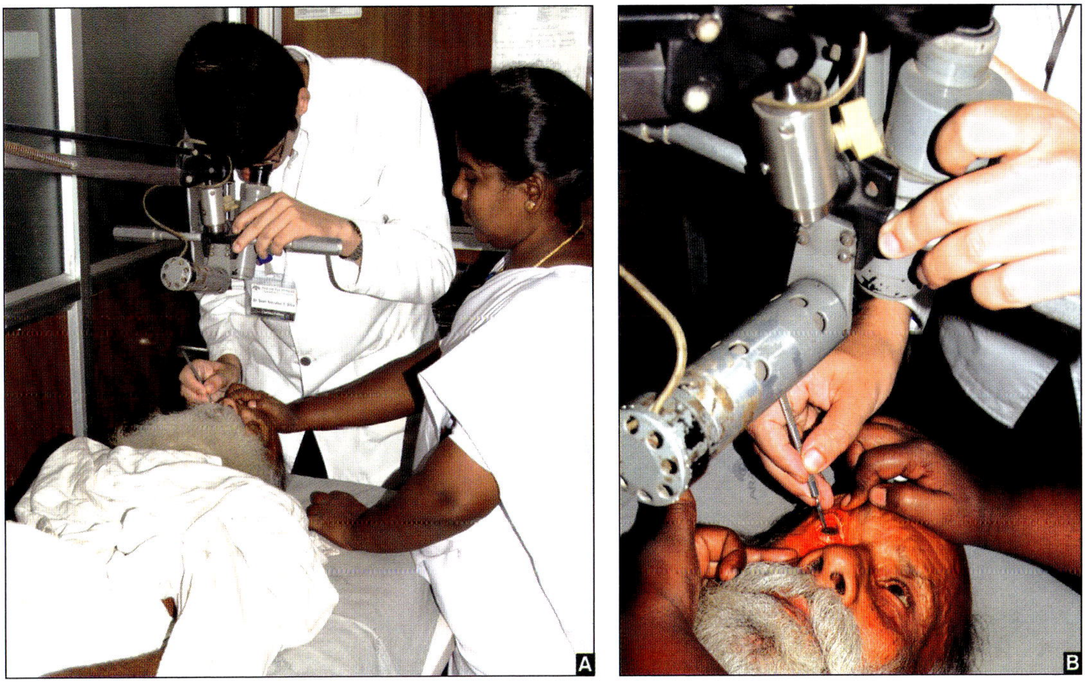

Figs 3.4A and B: Corneal scraping collected by an ophthalmologist by using ophthalmic microscope

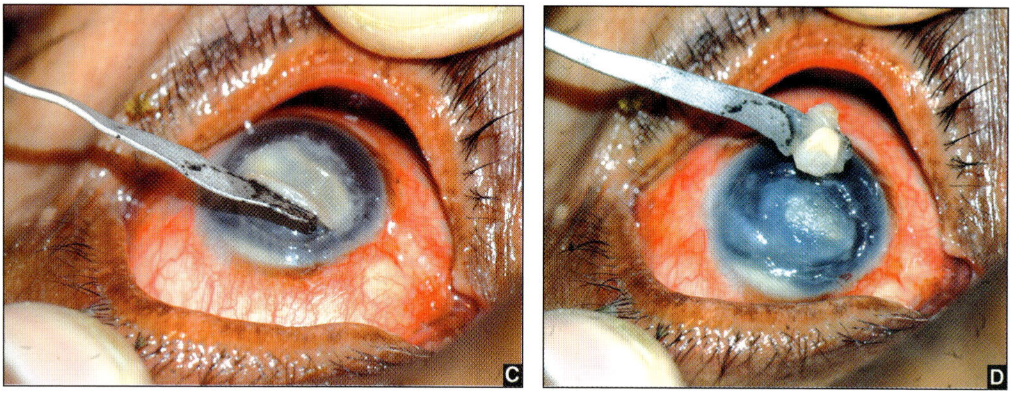

Figs 3.4C and D: Infected area gently scraped by using Kimura's spatula. Scrapping helps to debulk the fungal load as in this case

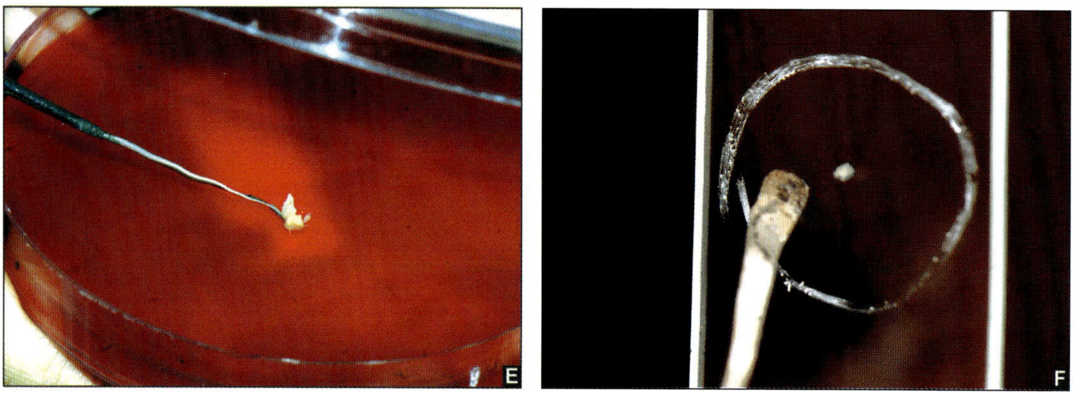

Figs 3.4E and F: Scraped material inoculated on Blood agar in multiple C streaks form (E) and smeared on a clean glass slide (F)

CHAPTER

4

Staining Procedure for Rapid Identification of Fungi

Scrapings from involved ocular site complemented with the appropriate staining method can offer the ophthalmologist circumstantial as well as definitive information concerning the identity of the invading organism.

STAINING METHODS

Light Microscopy

- KOH
- Gram's stain
- Giemsa stain
- Grocott-Gomori Methenamine Silver (GMS) stain.

Fluorescent Microscopy

- Calcofluor white staining
- KOH-Calcofluor white procedure.

KOH mount

Principle: Potassium hydroxide is used as a mounting fluid for visualization of fungal filaments as it helps in the clearance or lyses of all surrounding tissues. In addition, *Acanthamoeba* cysts and *Nocardia* filaments can also be visualized.

Preparation of 10% KOH

- Approximately 1 gm (8 pellets) of KOH is weighed
- It is dissolved in 10 ml of distilled water
- One drop of 10% glycerol is added
- Fresh stock should be prepared every week
  Can be kept at room temperature in a dropper bottle like a penicillin bottle (Fig. 4.1).

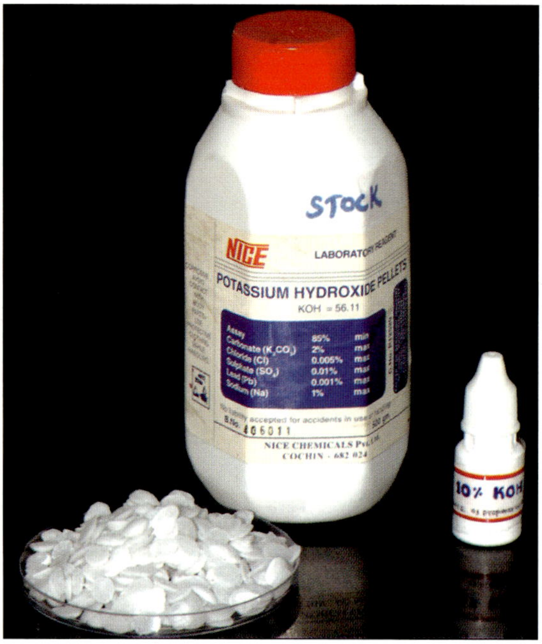

Fig. 4.1: KOH pellets and preparation of 10% KOH

Procedure

- Take a clean glass slide and place the sample on the center.
- Add a drop of 10% KOH and place a cover slip.
- Take special care to avoid any air bubbles.
- Observe under low and high power.

Interpretation

Fungal filaments: Appear as refractile hyphae with septate or aseptate, branching filaments or non-branching filaments. Some filaments look brown in color due to melanin pigments in their cell wall as in some species of dematiaceous fungi. It is however, not possible to identify the species of fungi from the wet mount.

Different morphological forms of fungal filaments from corneal scraping specimen (Figs 4.2 to 4.8).

Yeast cells are oval or round and colorless and may at times produce pseudohyphae in the KOH wet mount preparation (Care should be taken to differentiate them from epithelial cells) (Fig. 4.9).

Nocardia filaments are slender, branching and much thinner in size when compared to fungal hyphae.

Acanthamoeba cysts in the KOH wet mount are typical star or hexagonal shaped and double cell walled structures (Care should be taken to differentiate them from epithelial cells).

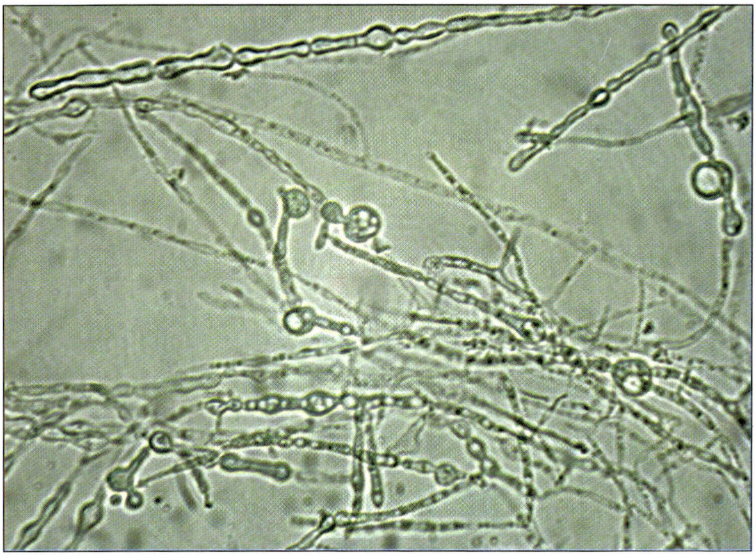

Fig. 4.2: Hyaline, septate fungal filaments in 10% KOH wet mount of corneal scraping specimen (400 X magnification)

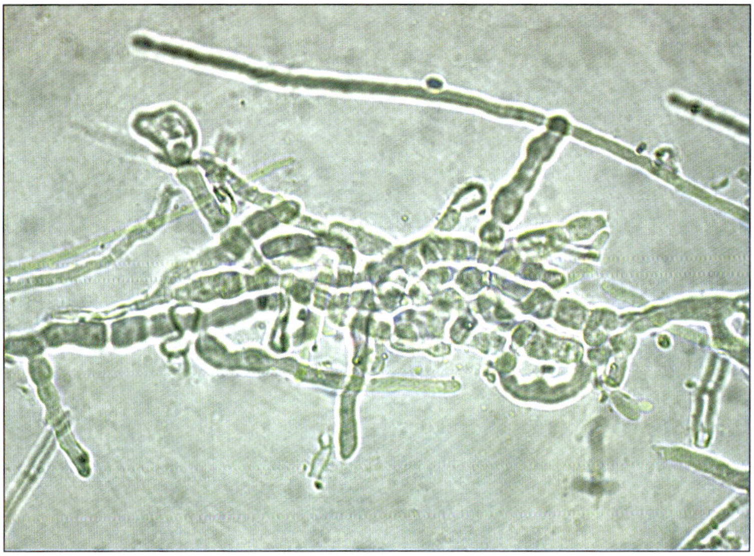

Fig. 4.3: Hyaline, septate, large, branching fungal filaments of corneal scraping in 10% KOH wet mount (400 X magnification)

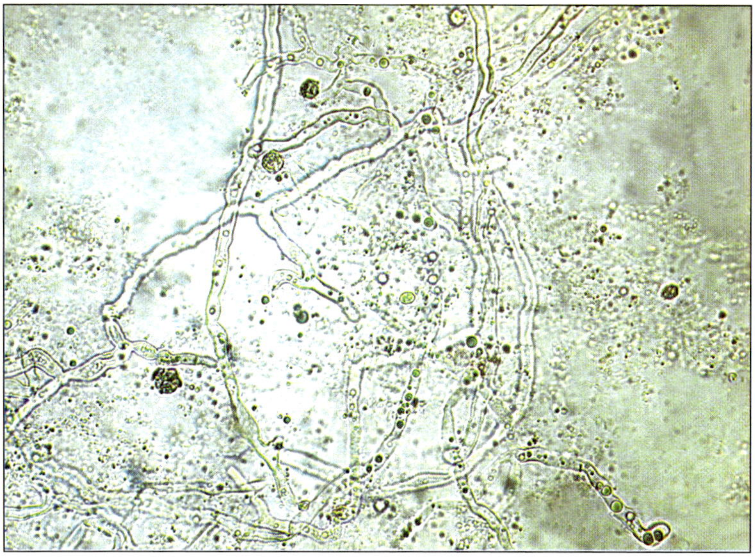

Fig. 4.4: Hyaline fungal filaments in KOH wet mount (400 X magnification)

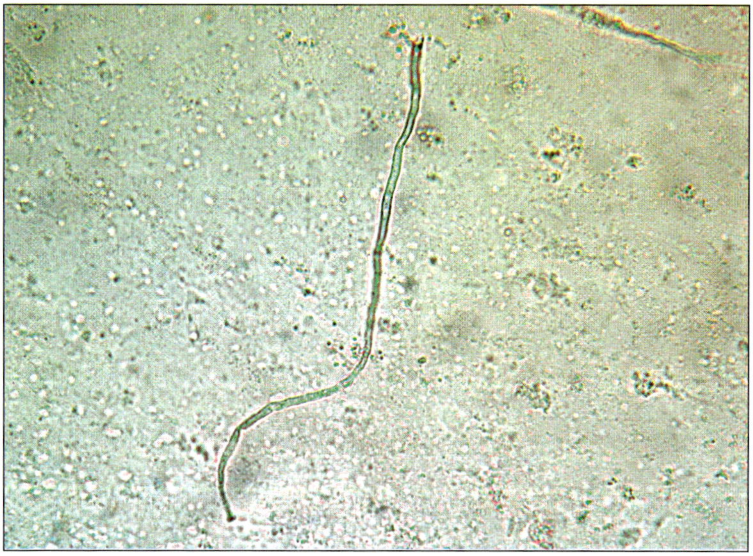

Fig. 4.5: Hyaline, septate fungal filament in KOH wet mount of aqueous fluid (400 X magnification)

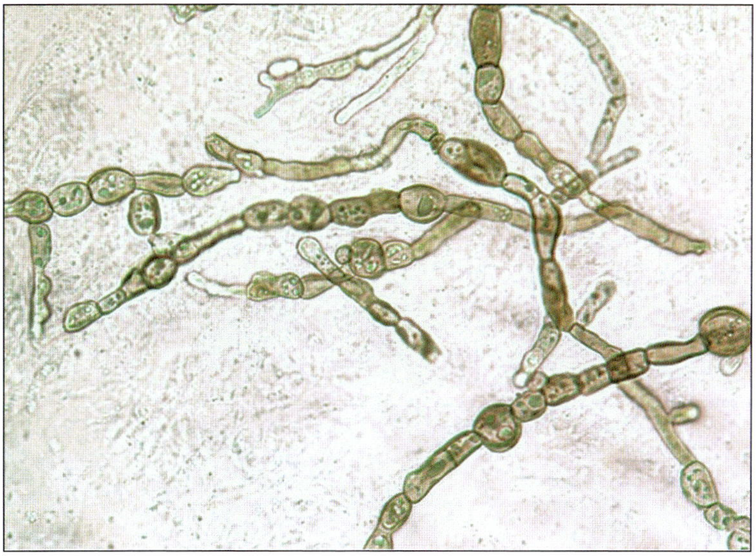

Fig. 4.6: Pigmented, septate fungal filaments in KOH wet mount of corneal scrapings. Culture grew Curvularia (400 X magnification)

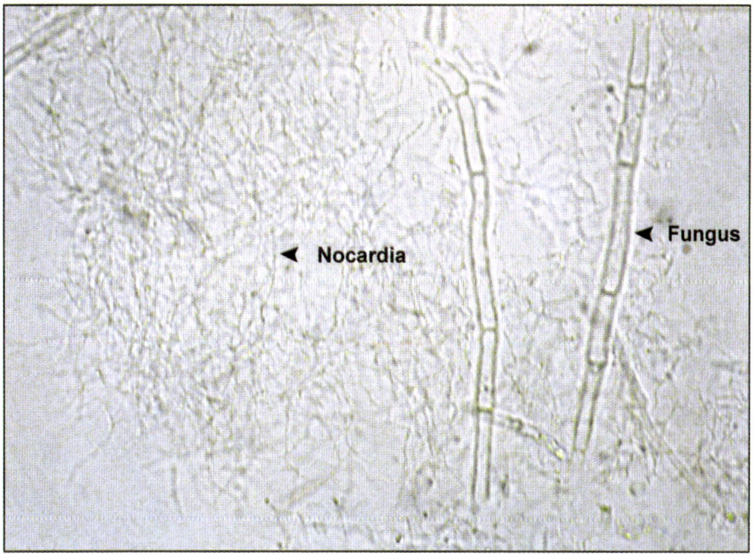

Fig. 4.7: A KOH mount showing hyaline septate fungal filaments and thin *Nocardia* filaments (isolated from a patient with corneal ulcer caused by mixed infections involving fungi and *Nocardia*)—(400 X magnification)

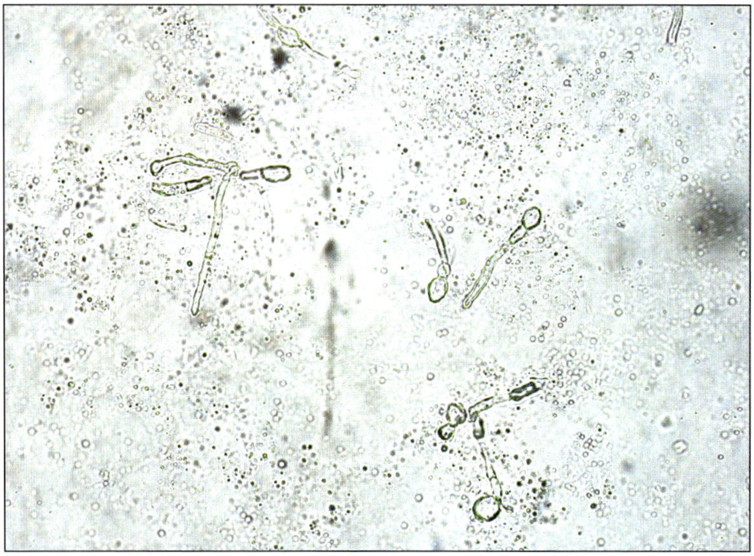

Fig. 4.8: Thin broken fungal filaments from a corneal ulcer under antifungal treatment (400 X magnification)

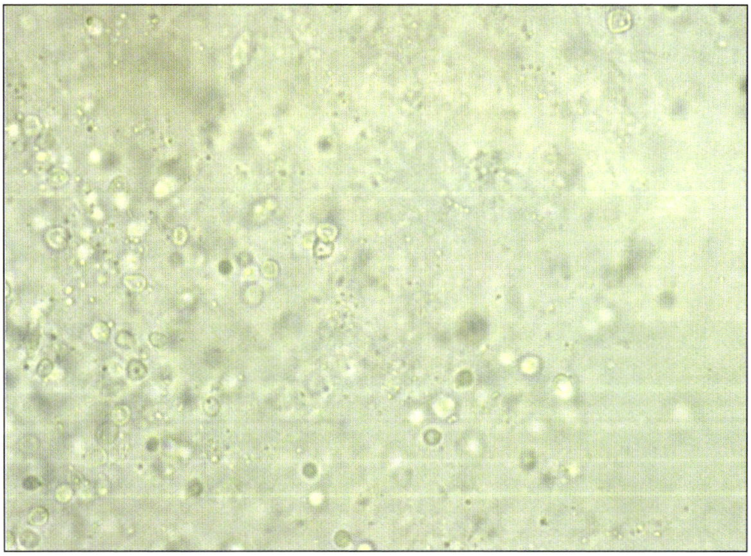

Fig. 4.9: Oval shaped yeast cells in KOH wet mount (400 X magnification)

Gram's Stain

Principle: Gram's staining is employed to distinguish and differentiate the type of infecting organism. The procedure requires application of four reagents in a sequential manner namely, a basic pararosaniline, an aqueous solution of iodine, a decolorizing solvent and pink counter stain. The violet dye and iodine combine to form an insoluble, dark purple compound in the bacterial protoplasm and cell wall. This compound is dissociable by the decolorizer, which dissolves and removes the components from the cell, the removal being much slower from gram-positive than from gram-negative bacteria. Gram-positive have thicker and dense peptidoglycon layers in thin cell walls, which makes them more permeable to the primary stain than the gram-negative bacteria. The iodine has a critical role in enhancing this difference. The organism is considered as gram-positive, if it appears violet under the microscope and gram-negative, if it appears pink under the microscope.

Procedure

- Prepare a thin smear of the specimen, dry in air and fix the smear by gentle heating over a Bunsen burner flame.
- Flood the slide with Gram's crystal violet for 1 minute.
- Wash with distilled water and flood the slide with Gram's iodine for 1 minute.
- Wash with distilled water
- The smear is decolorized with acetone – alcohol solution and wash immediately (important to be careful in this step as too much decolorizing will show gram-positive as negative and vice versa)
- Wash with distilled water and counter stain with carbol fuchsin for 30 seconds.
- Wash with water, dry and examine the slide under oil immersion.

Note: Decolorizer is prepared by adding equal volumes of acetone and isopropanol. Cedar wood oil or liquid paraffin may be used. The components of Gram's stain are readily available in laboratory supplies stores (Fig. 4.10).

Interpretation

Fungus: **Filamentous fungi** have varying staining response to Gram's stain They either do not stain at all or may stain gram-positive or gram-negative. However, this method is also useful for identifying any coexisting bacterial infection. **Gram-positive bacteria** appear purple (blue) in color and may be either cocci or bacilli. **Gram-negative bacteria** appear pink – red in color and may be either cocci or bacilli. ***Nocardia*** is a thin gram positive branching beaded filaments. **Yeasts** are gram-positive (purple), round or oval shaped (Figs 4.11 to 4.18).

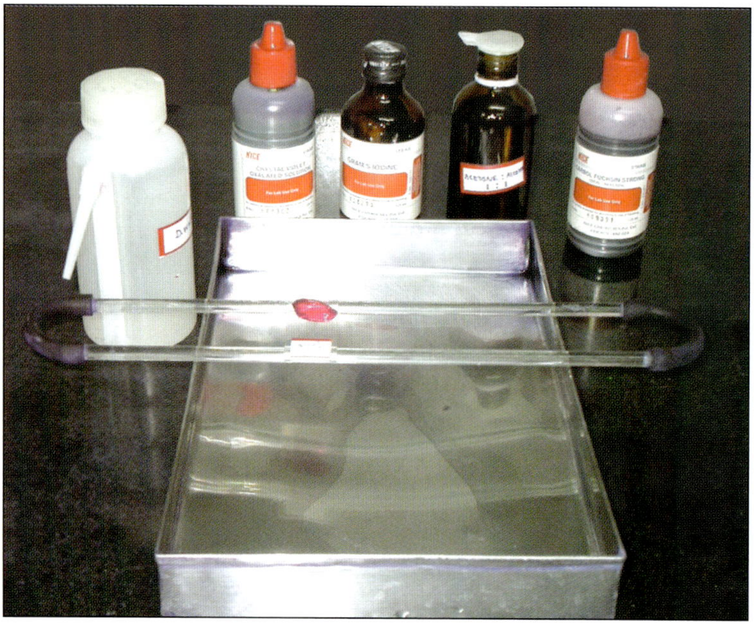

Fig. 4.10: Gram's stain kit

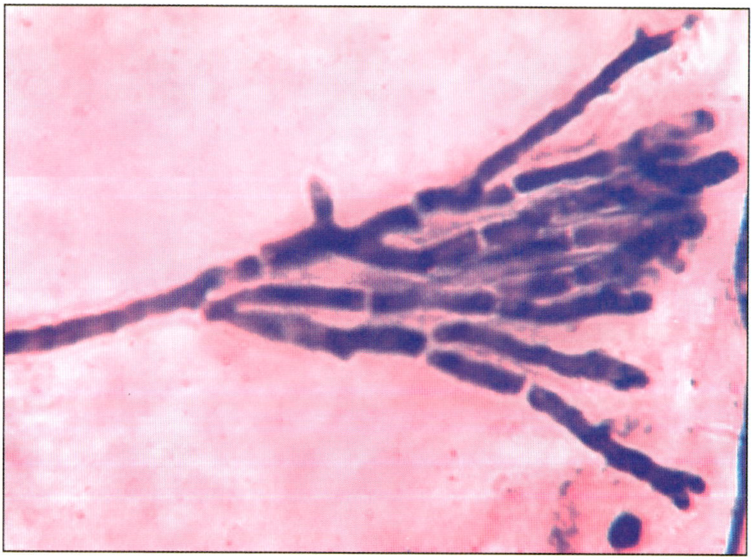

Fig. 4.11: Gram's stain showing branching fungal filaments from corneal scraping (1000 X magnification)

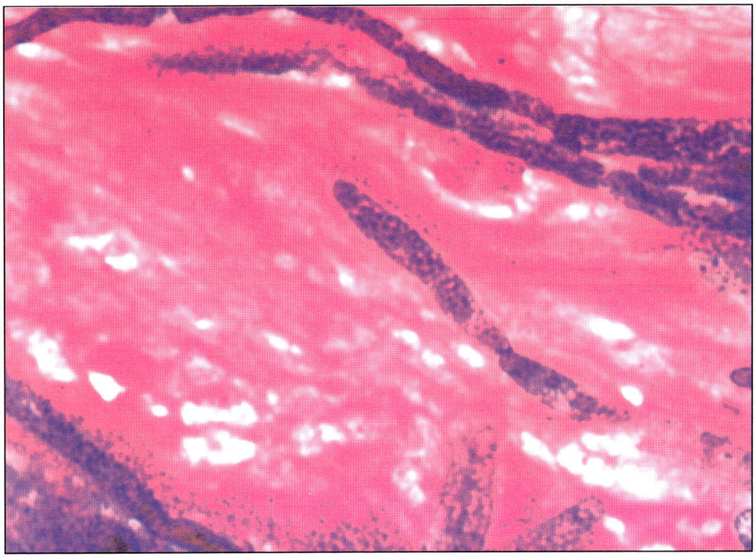

Fig. 4.12: Large fungal filaments stained with crystal violet of Gram staining (1000 X magnification)

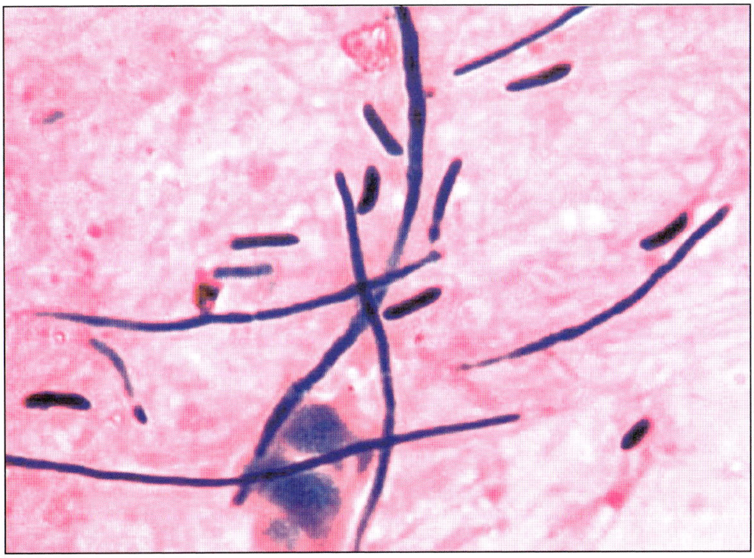

Fig. 4.13: Long fungal filaments with sickle shaped spores (morphologically resembles *Fusarium* spp) from corneal ulcer cases (1000 X magnification)

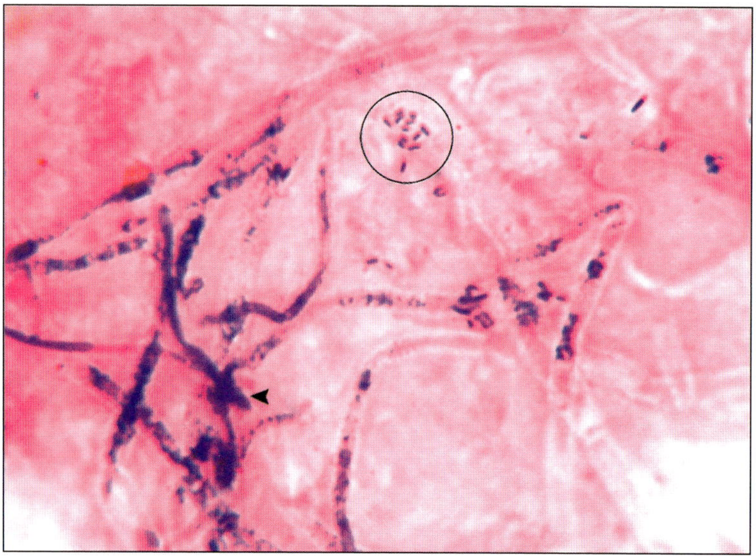

Fig. 4.14: A Gram's stain slide picture showing fungal filaments (➤) and gram-positive bacilli (isolated from a patient with corneal ulcer caused by mixed infections involving fungi and bacteria) (1000 X magnification)

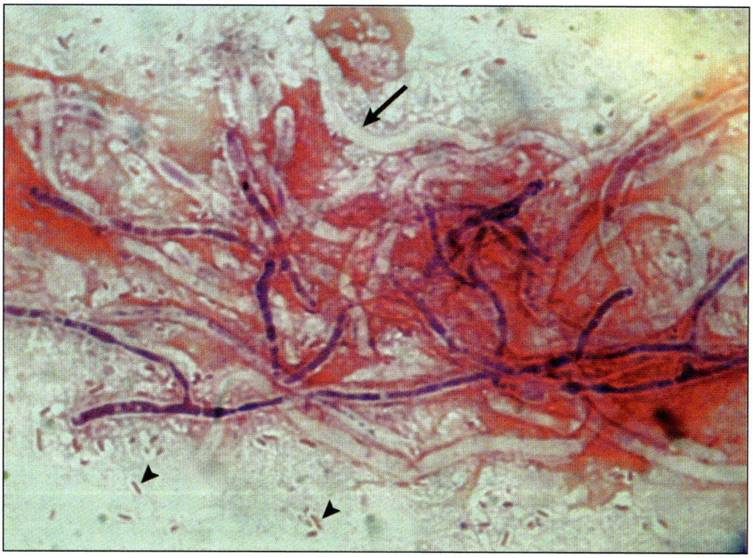

Fig. 4.15: A Gram stain slide picture showing fungal filaments and gram-negative bacilli (➤) (isolated from a patient with corneal ulcer caused by a mixed infections involving fungi and bacteria) (1000 X magnification)

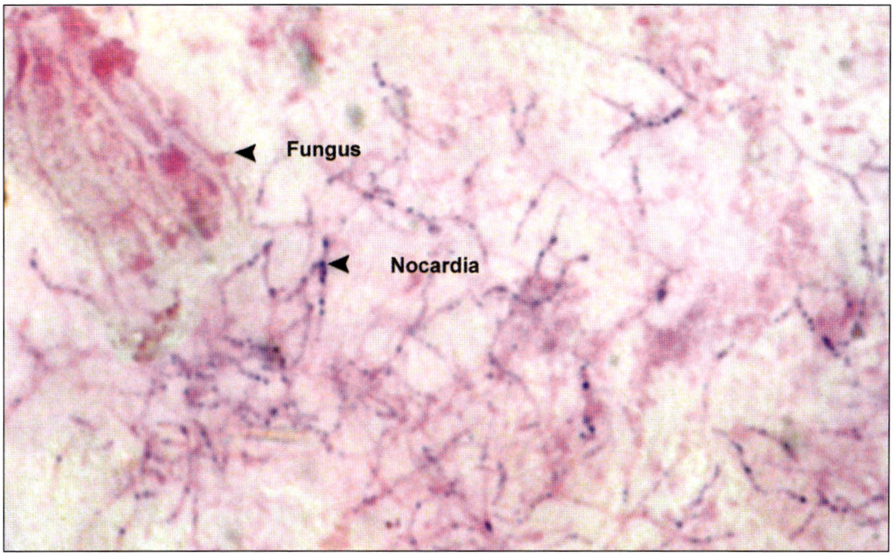

Fig. 4.16: A Gram stain slide picture showing fungal filaments and gram-positive beaded filaments of *Nocardia* (isolated from a patient with corneal ulcer caused by mixed infections involving fungi and *Nocardia*) (1000 X magnification)

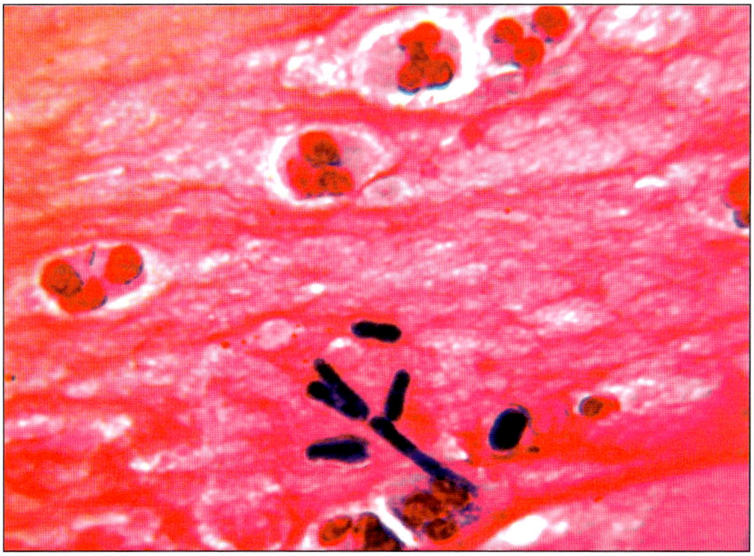

Fig. 4.17: A Gram stain slide picture from corneal scrapping showing gram-positive budding yeast cells of *Candida* spp (1000 X magnification)

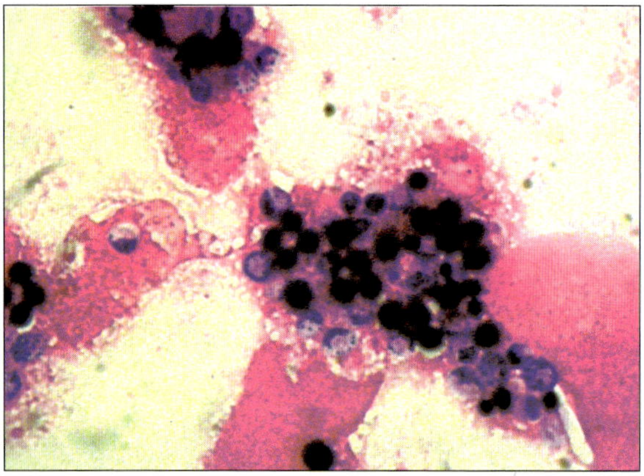

Fig. 4.18: A Gram stain slide picture from corneal scrapping showing clumps of gram-positive yeast cells (100 X magnification)

Grocott-Gomori Methenamine Silver (GMS) Stain

Principle: To detect positive fungal elements, which, after staining take on a silver or black color. The light green counter stain is used to stain the background a contrasting color. Hematoxylin may also be used.

Preparation

Materials and reagents for the Gomori methanamine silver stain

1. Gelatin – coated glass slides (stored at – 20° C to 0 °C)
2. Chromic acid solution 5%
3. Methenamine silver nitrate solution:
   a. Methenamine, 3% : 100 ml
   b. Silver nitrate, 0.1% : 7 ml
4. Gold chloride, 0.1%
5. Sodium thiosulfate solution, 2%
6. Stock light green solution:
   a. Light green, SF : 0.2 gm
   b. Distilled water : 100 ml
   c. Glacial acetic acid : 0.2 ml
7. Absolute methyl alcohol
8. Distilled water.

Procedure

- Fix slide in absolute methyl alcohol for 5 minutes
- Oxidize in 5% chromic acid for 30 minutes
- Immerse in preheated methenamine silver nitrate solution for 20 minutes
- Wash with six changes of distilled water
- Tone for 2 to 4 minutes in 0.1% gold chloride
- Rinse with two changes of distilled water
- Immerse in 2% sodium thiosulfate solution for 2 minutes
- Wash with tap water

- Counter stain for 1 minute with fresh 1: 5 dilution in distilled water of stock light green solution
- Air dry, clean and mount.
- Examine by light microscopy using 400X and 1000X magnification

Interpretation: Fungal elements stain silver to black, using a low power objective; fungal elements can easily be seen in a tissue section (Fig. 4.19). *Acanthamoeba* cell walls stain silver, Microsporidia stain primarily silver and then only if the cell wall is intact.

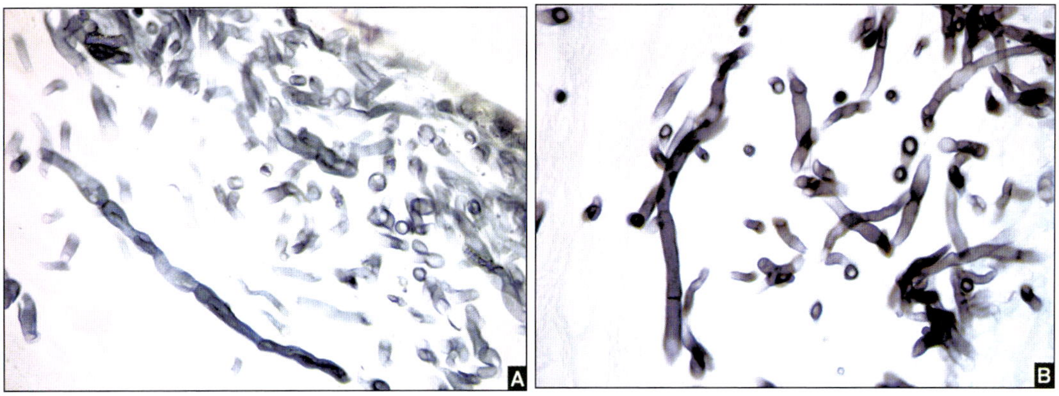

Figs 4.19A and B: Fungal elements stain silver to black in Gomori methenamine silver (GMS) stain – Tissue biopsy (400 X magnification)

Fluorescent Microscopy

Calcofluor White Staining

Purpose: Calcofluor white stain is a rapid staining procedure used to detect fungi, *Acanthamoeba* cysts, or Microsporidia spores in smears from clinical specimens.

Principle: Calcofluor white binds to β1 – 3, β1 – 4 polysaccharides such as cellulose, and chitin, and fluoresces bright apple-green when exposed to long-wavelength ultraviolet light or short wavelength visible light. Cell walls of fungi contain large amounts of chitin, and therefore yeast cells, hyphae, and pseudohyphae are readily visualized. Nonspecific staining of *Acanthamoeba* cysts and spores of Microsporidia also has been observed.

Procedure

1. Fix slide in methanol for 3 to 5 minutes.
2. Add several drops of solution prepared as follows: combine equal amounts of 0.1% Calcofluor white stain and 0.1% Evans blue dissolved in distilled water
3. After 5 minutes remove excess stain and apply a cover slip
4. Examine using a fluorescence microscope for characteristic apple-green (or red if filter is used) chemo fluorescence of fungi and amoebic cysts. We used a Nikon fluorescence microscope with orange-red filter.

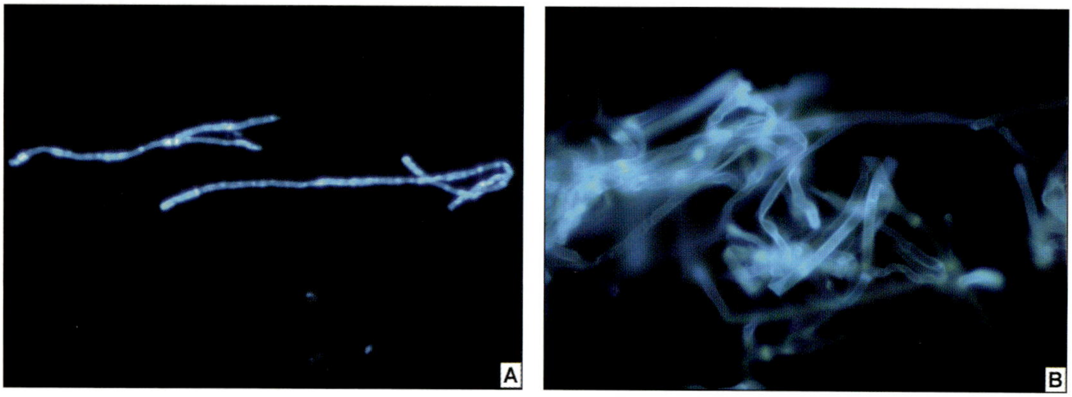

Figs 4.20A and B: Blue white fluorescence of fungal hyphae of corneal scraping in KOH Calcofluor staining (**A** – 200 X magnification, **B** – 400 X magnification)

Interpretation

1. Positive fluorescence is apple-green (or bright orange-red if filter is used) (Fig. 4.20).
2. Background and other cells stain red-brown.

Potassium Hydroxide – Calcofluor White Procedure

Purpose: CFW combining with KOH for enhanced detection of fungi in clinical specimens

Principle: KOH in solution with Calcofluor white, a fluorescent brightener of textiles, enhances the visualization of fungal elements in microscopic specimens. Calcofluor white binds to both chitin and cellulose in fungal cell walls and fluoresces bright green to blue.

Preparation

1. 15% Potassium Hydroxide solution
   Water (distilled) ....80 ml
   KOH ....15 gm
   Glycerol ....20 ml
   Dissolve KOH in water and glycerol.
   Store at 25°C, and re-prepare if a precipitate forms.
2. 0.1% (wt/vol) Calcofluor white solution
   Water (distilled)............. 1000 ml
   Calcofluor white stain...... 1 gm
   Mix, heating gently, if precipitate develops (or filter if persistent). Store in the dark at room temperature.

Procedure

1. Place specimen on clean glass slide
2. Add a drop of each solution (15% KOH and Calcofluor white)
3. Mix and cover with glass cover slip.
4. Allow to sit at room temperature until material is clear (warming slide will hasten process).
5. Examine using a fluorescence microscope with 10X and 40X to 50X objective or 100X oil.

Interpretation: Fungi stain bright green or blue-white, depending on the filter.

CHAPTER

5

Recommendations for Isolation of Fungi from Ocular Specimens

RECOMMENDED MEDIA FOR FUNGI ISOLATION

Clinical specimens are processed promptly and plated to isolation media as a means to recover fungi that may be causing disease. Media and incubation temperatures are selected to allow for the growth of pathogenic and opportunistic yeasts and fungi.

Isolation Media

The following Table is intended as a guideline for media required for the primary isolation of common isolates in ocular infections. Because some of these sites may be sterile sources and others are nonsterile sources, isolates considered pathogenic differ by site.

Media and smears to be inoculated for received swabs and aspiration fluids				
Source/site	*Routine media*	*Anaerobe*	*Fungal*	*AFB*
Eyelid	BA, CA	If requested	PDA	---
Conjunctiva	BA, CA	If requested	PDA	--
Lacrimal	BA, CA, BHI, Thio	Anaerobic Blood agar	PDA, LJ	LJ
Abscess or drainage	BA, CA, BHI, Thio	Anaerobic Blood agar	PDA	LJ
Cornea	BA, CA, BHI, Thio	Anaerobic Blood agar	PDA	LJ
Vitreous, aqueous	BA, CA, BHI, Thio	*	PDA / LJ	LJ
Donor cornea rim and MK media	BA, CA, Thio			

* Anaerobic cultures are performed on intraocular fluids wherever necessary.

Media abbreviated as follows:

BA : Blood agar
CA : Chocolate blood agar
BHI : Brain heart infusion broth
Thio : Thioglycolate broth culture
SDA : Sabouraud's dextrose agar (Emmons modification)
LJ : Lowenstein jensen agar slant
BHI : Brain heart infusion broth

A variety of media are available for the primary inoculation and recovery of fungi from clinical specimens. No one specific medium or combination of media is adequate for all specimens. Media must be carefully selected based on specimen type and fungal suspected agents. Media is dispensed into bottles or 100 mm Petri dishes. Petri plates offer the advantage of a large surface area for isolation and dilution of inhibitory substances in the specimens, but must be poured thick with at least 25 ml of medium to resist dehydration during incubation. Because plates are vented, they are more likely to become contaminated during incubation. Each Petri plate must be labeled on the bottom, and the lid must be taped at two points to prevent accidental opening of the plate. All inoculated media should be read every day initially following incubation. Plates must be opened only within a biological safety cabinet to prevent contamination of the plate and exposure of personnel to potentially dangerous fungi.

Media in bottles have a smaller surface area but offer maximum safety and resistance to dehydration and contamination. If the specimen is from a contaminated site, it is important to include media that contain inhibitory substances such as chloramphenicol, gentamicin or cycloheximide. Chloramphenicol or gentamicin will inhibit most bacterial contaminants, while cycloheximide inhibits most saprobic moulds. It is important to remember that Cycloheximide may also inhibit opportunistic fungi such as some species of *Aspergillus*, *Fusarium*, *Scopulariopsis*, *Pseudallescheria*, *Zygomycetes*, some dematiaceous fungi, and yeasts such as *Cryptococcus* neoformans and some *Candida* species.

Antibacterial agents may inhibit the growth of aerobic *Actinomycetes* like *Nocardia* sp. It is important to use media with and without inhibitory agents. Specimens from normally sterile sites can be inoculated to media without inhibitory substances.

Potato Glucose Agar (Potato Dextrose Agar)

Composition

Potatoes	200 gm
Glucose	10 gm
Agar	18 gm
Distilled water	1000 ml

Preparation

- Peel the potatoes, cut into cubes and boil in water for one hour
- Filter through cheesecloth, add glucose and agar; bring to a boil to dissolve agar completely and filter again on Whatman #2 filter paper.
- Adjust the volume to 1 liter
- Sterilize at 121°C for 15 minutes.

Quality Control

Appearance: Colorless or light yellow, solid medium, transparent or translucent
Final pH at 25°C: 5.6 ± 0.2

Sterility Check

One representative sample of the prepared culture plate is incubated at 25 - 30°C for 4 days to check the sterility of the media.

This medium is also available commercially.

Sabouraud's Dextrose Agar (SDA)

Principle

SDA agar formulation was originally described by Sabouraud for the cultivation of fungi. Emmons' modification contains 2% glucose and is slightly acidic (pH 6.5). It is the standard medium for recovery and maintenance of a wide variety of fungi commonly isolated in the clinical laboratory. The original SDA formulation specifies 4% glucose. Emmons' modification with less glucose is preferred as an isolation medium because some isolates, notably Blastomyces dermatitidis may not be recovered using the original Sabouraud's formulation. Peptone is the source of nitrogenous growth factors while dextrose provides an energy source for the growth of microorganisms.

a. SDA (acidic Ph)

Ingredients	*grams/liter of distilled water*
Dextrose	40
Peptone	10
Agar	20

Final pH: 5.5-5.6

b. SDA (neutral Ph-Emmon's modification)

Ingredients	*grams/liter of distilled water*
Dextrose	20
Peptone	18
Agar	20

Final pH: 6.8-7.0

c. Directions
   - Dissolve all the ingredients by boiling.
   - Dispense in plates and autoclave at 121°C for 15 minutes.
   - Adjust the final pH.
   - The tubes are cooled in a slanted position and stored in the refrigerator (4°C).

d. Quality control

Colour and clarity: Light amber colored. Clear to slightly opalescent gel.

Reaction: Reaction of the molten media is pH 6.8-7

Cultural response:
- Cultural characteristics after 48-72 hr at 30°C.
- *Candida albicans* will produce luxuriant growth

Sterility check: One representative sample of the prepared culture plate is incubated at 25-30°C for 4 days to check the sterility of the media.

Brain-heart Infusion Agar (BHI)

Principle

It is a highly nutritious medium that can support the growth of wide variety of microorganisms. It can be further enriched by the addition of blood or rendered selective by adding different antibiotics. BHI is an enriched medium that enhances the recovery of *Cryptococcus neoformans* from sterile specimens such as CSF. BHI is also used in yeast-mould conversions for *Sporothrix* and *Paracoccidioides*.

Ingredients	*gms/liter*
Calf brain infusion	200
Beef heart infusion	250
Peptone	10
Dextrose	2.00
Sodium chloride	5.00
Disodium phosphate	2.50
Agar	15

Final pH (at 25°C): 7.4 ± 0.2

Directions

- Dissolve ingredients by boiling
- Dispense in bottles and sterilize by autoclaving at 15lbs pressure for 15 minutes.

Quality Control

Sterility

Cultural response: Cultural characteristics after 48-72 hrs at 30°C.

Organisms	*Growth*
Cryptococcus neoformans	Luxuriant

CHAPTER

6

Incubation and Processing of Cultures in the Laboratory

Once the specimen has been inoculated on the media by the ophthalmologist, and received in the microbiology laboratory, the plates and tubes or broths must be placed in the appropriate atmosphere and temperature for isolation. Occasionally it is necessary to process specimens that are not set up at the bedside but are submitted to the microbiology laboratory on swabs or in syringes. Given below is the description for processing of specimens for fungal cultures.

INCUBATION REQUIREMENTS

Conditions (Fig. 6.1)

Temperature: 25°C to 30°C

Atmosphere: Sabouraud's dextrose agar or potato dextrose agar for fungi is incubated in a regular non - CO_2 incubator.

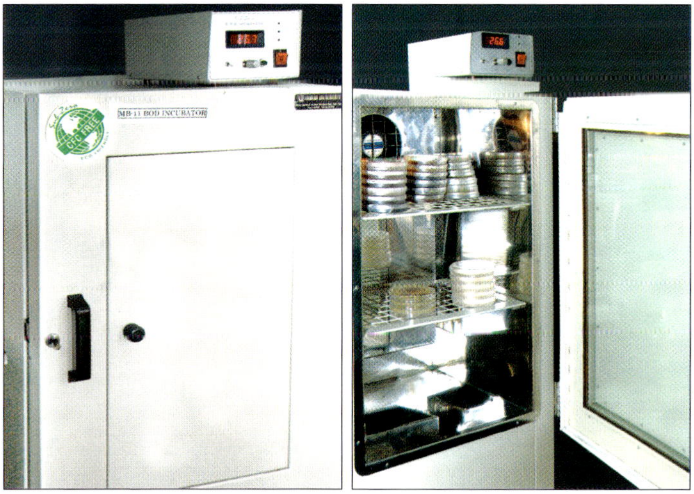

Fig. 6.1: Mycological incubator: Maintains temperature at 26°C

Length of Incubation: 7 days to 21 days, but varies depending on the specimen and or culture.

PROCESSING OF CULTURES

Fungal Cultures (Fig. 6.2)

Fungal plates/tubes are to be observed daily for the first week, because *Aspergillus* spp may be positive within 24 to 48 hours, as may *Fusarium* spp the two most common causes of mycotic keratitis. Significant growth (i.e., all fungi growing in the inoculated area of the agar or true pathogen) should be immediately informed to the physician with a written preliminary report and with the note "Final report to follow."

Cultures showing no growth should be followed by a written report at 7 days and final report "No growth" at 3 weeks. Lacto phenol cotton blue wet preparations are recommended for initial observation of fungi for spores.

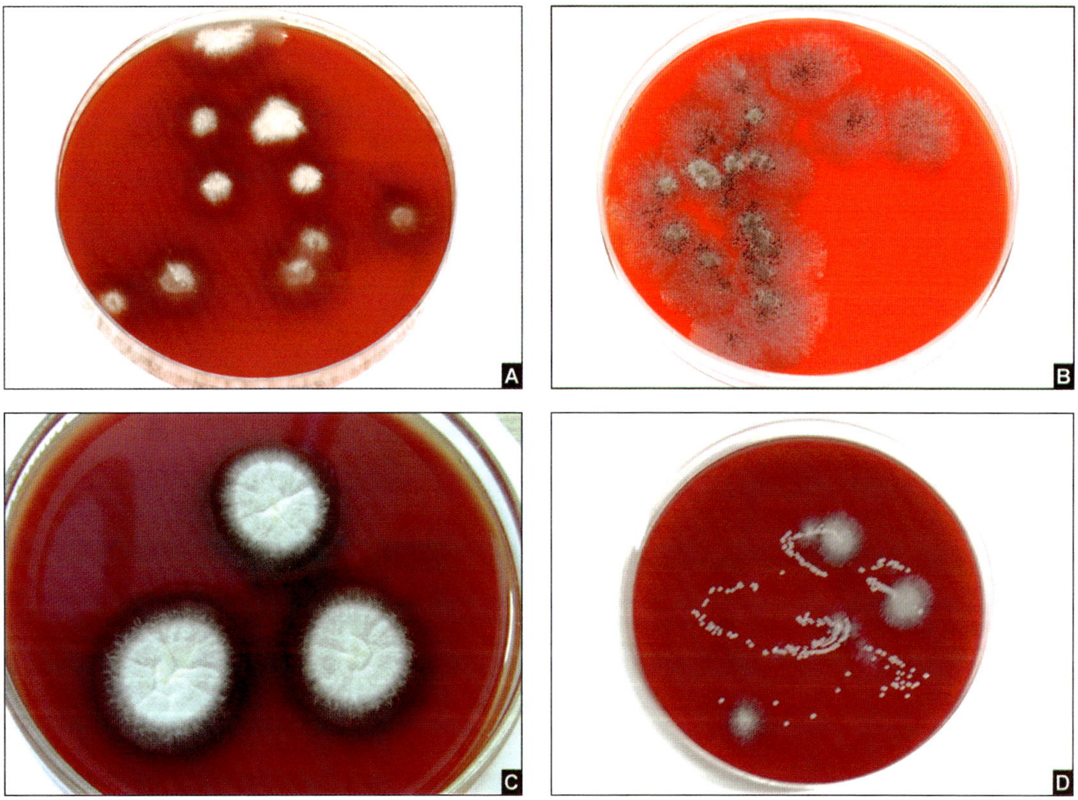

Figs 6.2A to D: Various form of fungal growth in blood agar of corneal scraping specimen culture. **A.** Profuse growth of hyaline fungus in all C streaks. **B.** Profuse growth of dematiaceous fungus in all C streaks. **C.** Growth of *A.flavus.* **D.** Mixed growth of fungus and bacteria

CHAPTER 7

Identification of Common Ocular Fungal Isolates

TECHNIQUES USED FOR MOULD IDENTIFICATION

Colony Characteristics

- To evaluate colony characteristics of filamentous fungi, it is necessary to subculture the fungus to the same media that the original colony descriptions are based upon.
- Visual examination of the colony will rapidly reveal important data concerning color, texture, diffusible pigments, exudates, growth zones, aerial and submerged hyphae, growth rate, colony topography, and macroscopic structures such as ascocarps, pycnidia, sclerotia, sporodochia, and synnemata.

Lactophenol Mounts

Prepare a mount of the fungus in lactophenol within the biological safety cabinet.

Lactophenol Cotton Blue Mounting Media

a. **Formulation:**

Phenol (concentrated)	:	20.0 ml
Lactic acid	:	20.0 ml
Glycerol	:	40.0 ml
Cotton blue	:	0.05 gm
Distilled water	:	20.0 ml

b. **Preparation:**

i. Mix phenol, lactic acid, glycerol and water in a 250 ml screw cap bottle.
ii. For lacto-phenol cotton bluc, dissolve 0.05 gm of cotton blue in 20 ml of water. Then add phenol, lactic acid and glycerol. Store in a 250 ml screw cap bottle.

c. **Quality control:**

Appearance: Deep blue liquid, slightly viscous
Usage : A mounting medium for microscopic examination.
Caution : Avoid exposure to phenol vapors during use.

TECHNIQUES OF MICROSCOPIC EXAMINATION

Principle

The simplest technique consists in placing a fragment of the colony between a slide and cover slip. This approach is rapid and often adequate for identification. Delicate fungal structures, however, are often broken by this process, rendering identification difficult.

The *adhesive tape technique* assists in maintaining the integrity of fungal structures by fixing them on the adhesive surface of a piece of transparent (Not frosted) tape.

The *slide culture technique* consists in growing a micro colony of the fungus on a slide or on a cover slip. The developing fungal colony adheres to the surface of the glass and facilitates the observation of intact conidial structures.

Methods

Direct Examination of a Portion of the Colony

- With the aid of sterile needle, detach a small fragment of the colony to be identified and place it in a drop of lactophenol cotton blue
- Using two needles gently spread apart the material to be examined
- Cover the preparation with a cover slip and press gently to flatten the preparation
- Examine under microscope with low magnification and then under higher magnification.

Adhesive Tape Technique

- Cut a piece of adhesive cellulose tape and fold it back on itself with the adhesive side turned outward. To hold on to the ends of the loop, forceps may be useful
- Press the adhesive side of the tape onto the surface of the colony and pull it away. The aerial hyphae of the colony will remain glued on to the tape surface
- Place the tape in a drop of lacto phenol-cotton blue previously placed at the center of a glass slide
- Examine microscopically (Fig. 7.1).

Slide Culture Technique (Ridell's Method)/Title Case

- Place a bent, U-shaped glass rod in the bottom of a sterile petri plate or sterile wet cotton ball in two corners of petriplate. Place a clean, sterile slide on the glass rod and then place a block of medium at the center of this slide
- Inoculate the sides of the medium block with small pieces of the culture to be identified.
- Place a cover slip sterilized by rapid passage over a flame onto the block of medium
- Pipette around 5 ml of sterile water onto the bottom of the petri plate to ensure maintenance of humidity, and then close the petri plate
- Incubate at an optimal temperature, generally 25°C
- The slide may be taken out of the petri plate and examined under the microscope at regular intervals (once in 7 days) to determine whether sporulation has occurred

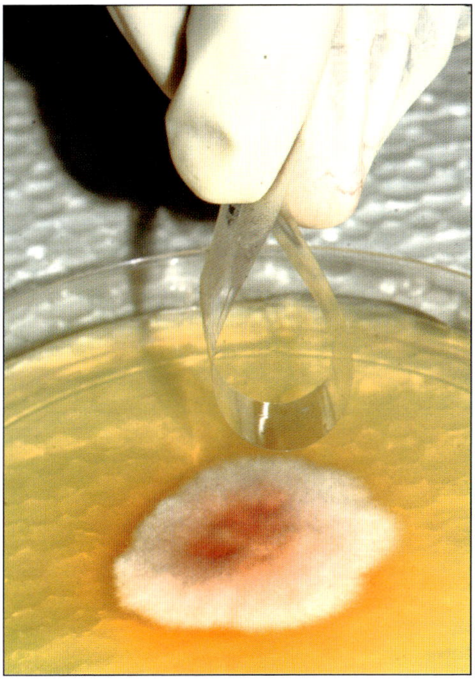

Fig. 7.1: Adhesive tape technique

- When the culture has sporulated, lift the cover slip from the medium block and fix it by passing it rapidly in close proximity to a burner flame. Mount it by placing it over a drop of cotton blue or other mounting fluid on a glass slide (Figs 7.2A to C)
- It is also possible to mount the portion of the culture which remains attached to the slide after disposing of the block of medium
- These preparations may be sealed by applying a layer of nail polish around the perimeter of the cover slip. Such preparations, if well sealed, may remain in good condition for 1-5 years.

Simplified Slide Culture Technique (Harris Method, Modified)

- Beginning with a petri plate of growth medium, cut two small blocks of medium from one side of the plate and place them on the surface of the medium near the opposite side
- Inoculate the sides of the two blocks with small pieces of the culture to be studied
- Place a cover slip sterilized by rapid passage through a flame onto each of the two blocks, close the petri plate, and incubate
- When appropriate, fix and mount the cover slips as described above.

REMARKS

When cover slips are being mounted, do not use more than a small quantity of mounting fluid between slide and cover slip. When the thickness of the preparation is minimized, most

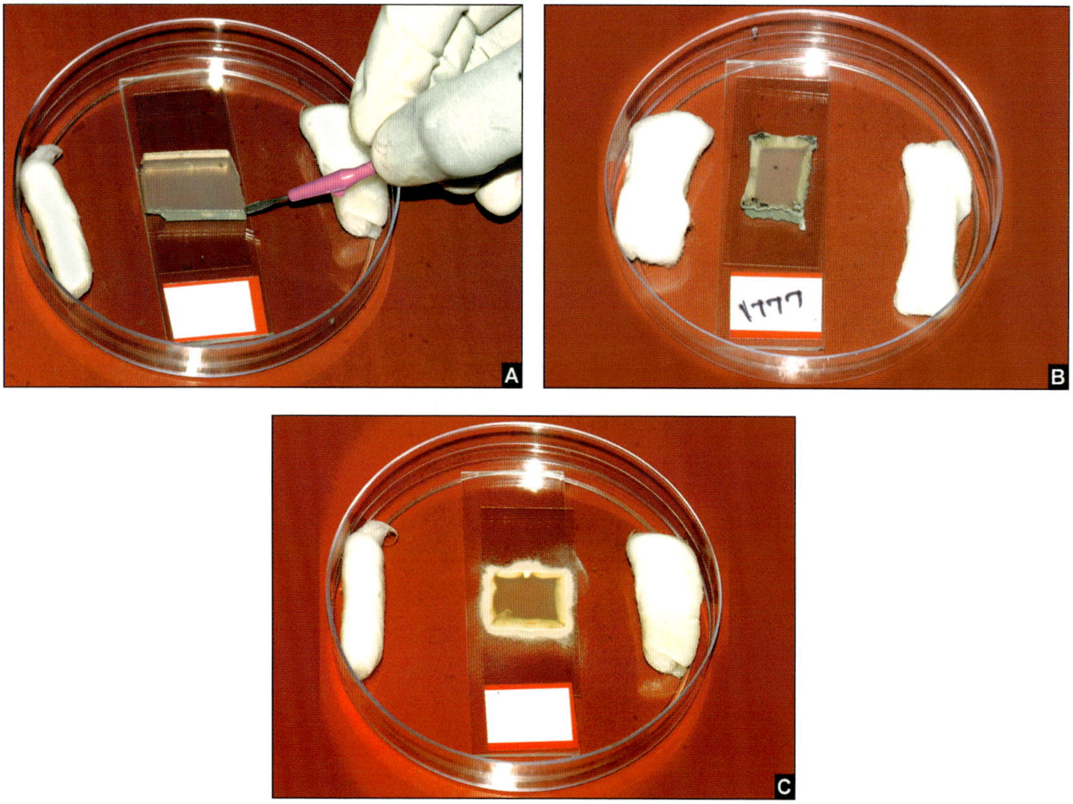

Figs 7.2A to C: Classic slide culture technique (Ridell's Method) **A.** Inoculation of fungal colony **B.** Dematiaceous fungus grown well after 5 days **C.** Well grown hyaline fungus ready to be observed for the morphological form

of the fungal structures will be in the same plane, making examination easier. This detail is especially important for photography. In addition, an excess of liquid will prevent proper sealing of the cover slip in any attempt to make a permanent mount of the preparation.

More enduring mounts can be produced by placing a small drop of lactophenol cotton blue on the cover slip bearing the fungal growth and covering it with a second cover slip of smaller size. This whole preparation is then placed with the smaller cover slip facing downward onto a drop of balsam or other permanent mounting material in the center of a slide.

CHAPTER

8

Macroscopic and Microscopic Characteristics of Ocular Fungal Isolates

ACREMONIUM

= *Cephalosporium* (Corda, 1839).

Pathogenicity

Acremonium

Acremonium has been reported as a rare cause of keratitis and endophthalmitis.

In the literature 17 cases of *Acremonium* keratitis have been reported between 1965 and 1991. Rosa et al (1994) found 3.2% of *Acremonium* keratitis in their series and Rodriguez-Ares et al reported this as an extremely rare cause of suppurative corneal infection.

Ecology

Cosmopolitan, isolated from soil and plant debris.

MACROSCOPIC MORPHOLOGY

- The growth rate of *Acremonium* colonies is moderately rapid, maturing within 5 days. The diameter of the colony is 1-3 cm following incubation at 25°C for 7 days on potato glucose agar.
- The texture of the colony is compact, flat or folded, and occasionally raised in the center. It is glabrous, velvety, and membrane-like at the beginning. Powdery texture may also be observed. By aging, the surface of the colony may become cottony due to the overgrowth of loose hyphae.
- The color of the colony is white, pale grey or pale pink on the surface. The reverse side is either uncolored or a pink to rose-colored pigment production is observed (Fig. 8.1).

MICROSCOPIC MORPHOLOGY

- *Acremonium* spp. possesses hyaline, septate hyphae which are typically very fine and narrow. Vegetative hyphae often form hyphal ropes. Unbranched, solitary, erect phialides are formed directly on the hyphal tips, the hyphal ropes, or both. The phialides are separated from hyphae by a septum and taper towards their apices. At the apices of the phialides is the hyaline conidia 2-3 × 4-8 µm in size. They usually appear in clusters, in balls or rarely as fragile chains.
- The conidia are bound by a gelatinous material. They may be single or multicellular, fusiform with a slight curve or resemble a shallow crescent. These structural properties of conidia vary depending on the species.
- *Acremonium falciforme* usually produces crescentic, nonseptate conidia. Sometimes, 2 or 3 celled conidia may also be observed. *Acremonium kiliense*, on the other hand, has short straight conidia and the conidia of *Acremonium recifei* are usually crescentic and nonseptate (Figs 8.1 and 8.2).

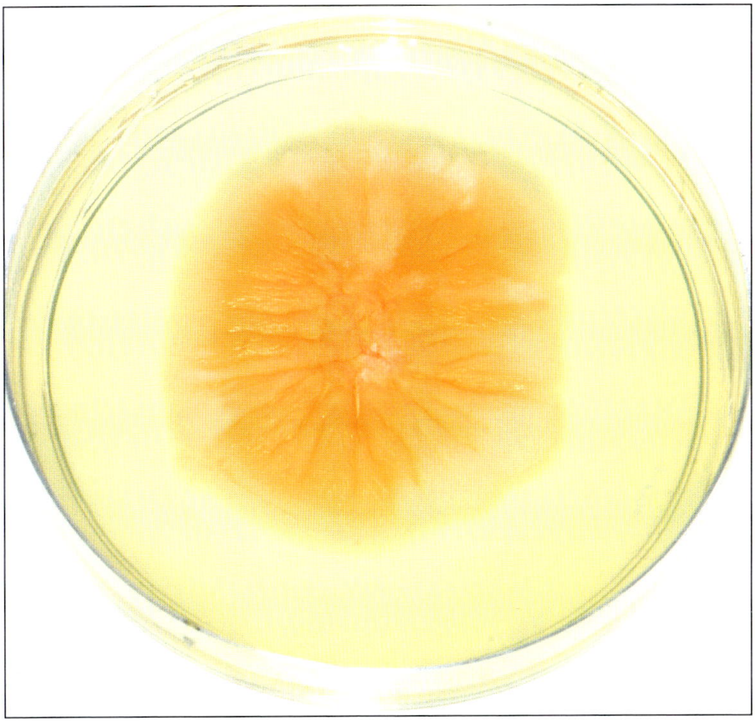

Fig. 8.1: *Acremonium* species on potato dextrose agar, 25°C, 7 days

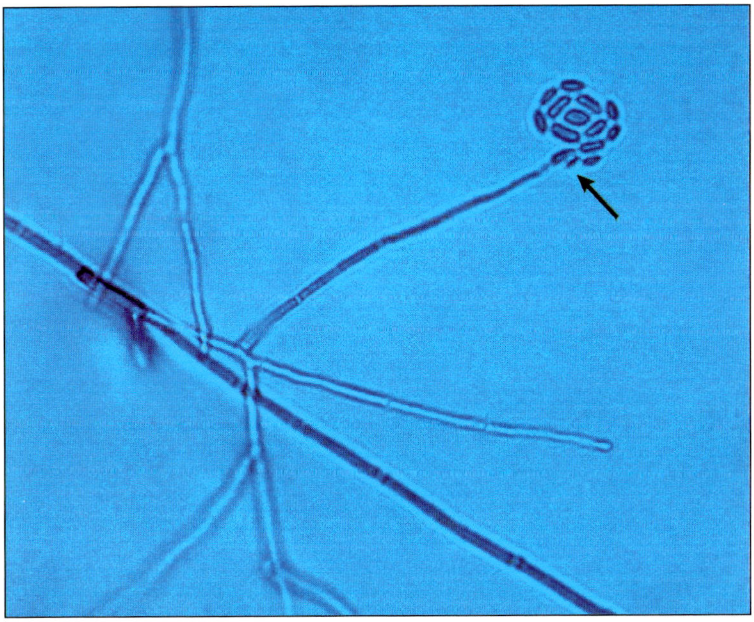

Fig 8.2: *Acremonium* species. Oblong conidia accumulating at the apices of narrow Phialides

ALTERNARIA

Pathogenicity

Occasional agents of keratitis, other infections include onychomycosis, ulcerated cutaneous infection, chronic sinusitis and rare cases of deep infection have also been reported in the immunocompromised patient.

Ecology

Alternaria is a cosmopolitan dematiaceous (phaeoid) fungus commonly isolated from plants, soil, food, and indoor air environment. The production of melanin-like pigment is one of its major characteristics.

MACROSCOPIC MORPHOLOGY

- *Alternaria* spp. grows rapidly and the colony size reaches a diameter of 3 to 9 cm following incubation at 25°C for 7 days on potato glucose agar (Fig. 8.3).
- The colony is flat, downy to woolly and is covered by grayish, short, aerial hyphae in time (Fig. 8.4).
- The surface is grayish white at the beginning which later darkens and becomes greenish black or olive brown with a light border.
- The reverse side is typically brown to black due to pigment production.

MICROSCOPIC MORPHOLOGY

- *Alternaria* spp. has septate, brown hyphae.
- Conidiophores are also septate and brown in color, occasionally producing a zigzag appearance. They bear simple or branched large conidia (7-10 × 23-34 μm) which have both transverse and longitudinal septations. These conidia may be observed singly or in acropetal chains and may produce germ tubes. They are ovoid to obclavate, darkly pigmented, muriform, and smooth or roughened.
- The end of the conidium nearest the conidiophores is round while it tapers towards the apex. This gives the typical beak or club-like appearance of the conidia.

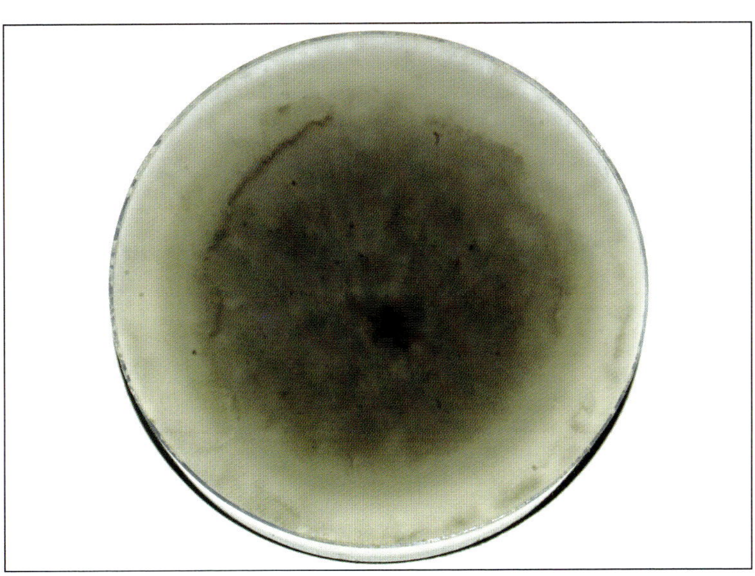

Fig. 8.3: *Alternaria* species. Growth on potato dextrose agar

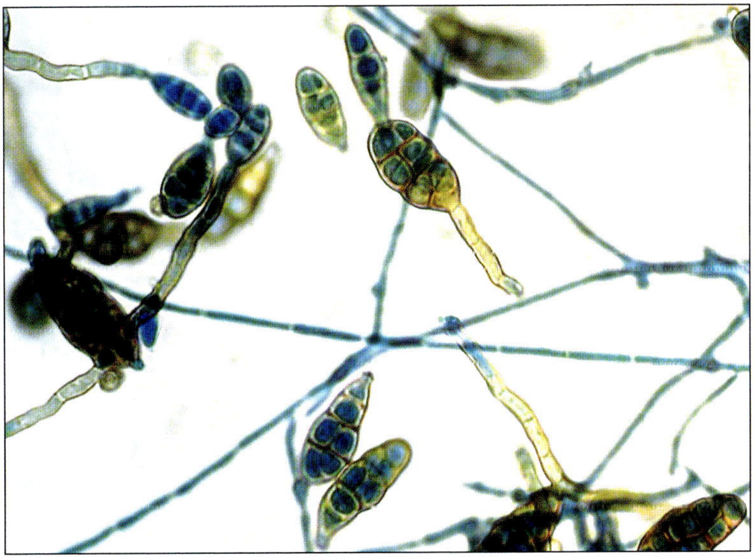

Fig. 8.4: *Alternaria* species. Obclavate, muriform conidia in chains

ASPERGILLUS SPECIES

Pathogenicity

At present, some twenty species of *Aspergillus* have been recognized as opportunistic pathogens. They are the most common cause of mycotic keratitis along with *Fusarium* spp.

Among all filamentous fungi, *Aspergillus* is in general the most commonly isolated in invasive infections. It is the second most commonly recovered fungus in opportunistic mycoses following *Candida*. Almost any organ or system in the human body may be involved. Onychomycosis, sinusitis, cerebral aspergillosis, meningitis, endocarditis, myocarditis, pulmonary aspergillosis, osteomyelitis, otomycosis, keratitis, endophthalmitis, cutaneous aspergillosis, hepatosplenic aspergillosis, as well as *Aspergillus* fungemia, and disseminated aspergillosis may develop.

Ecology

Aspergillus spp. abounds in the environment worldwide, thriving on a variety of substrates such as corn, decaying vegetation and soil. These fungi are also common contaminants in hospital air.

The color of the colony in various *Aspergillus* species is summarised in Table 8.1

Table 8.1: The color of the colony in various Aspergillus species

Species	*Surface*	*Reverse*	*Conidial head*
A. flavus	Yellow-green	Goldish to red-brown	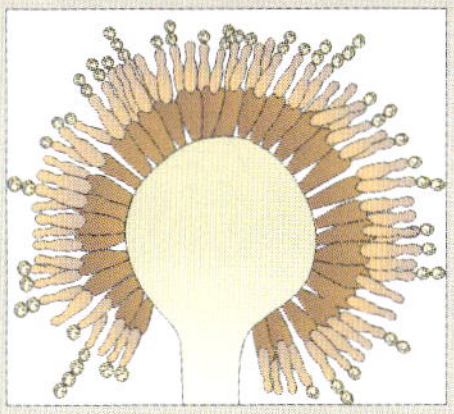
A. fumigatus	Blue-green to gray	White to tan	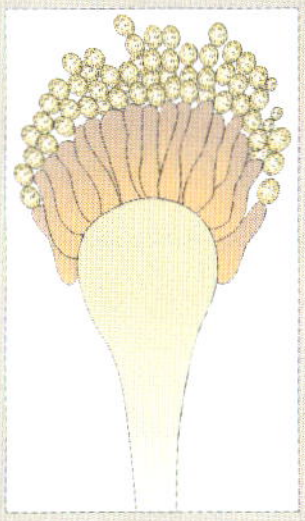
A. nidulans	Green, buff to yellow	Purplish red to olive	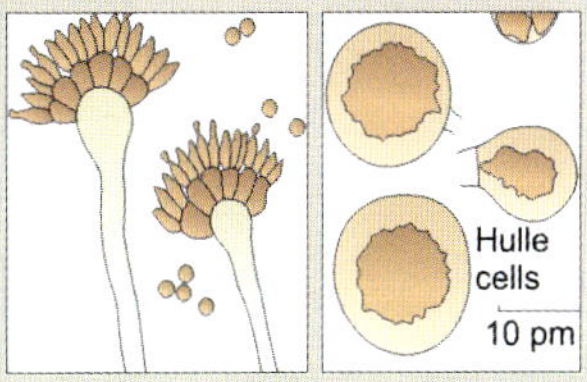
A. niger	Black	White to yellow	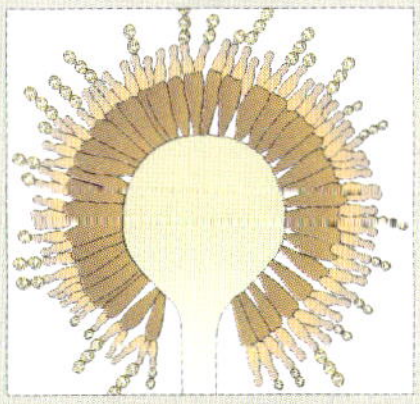
A. terreus	Cinnamon to brown	White to brown	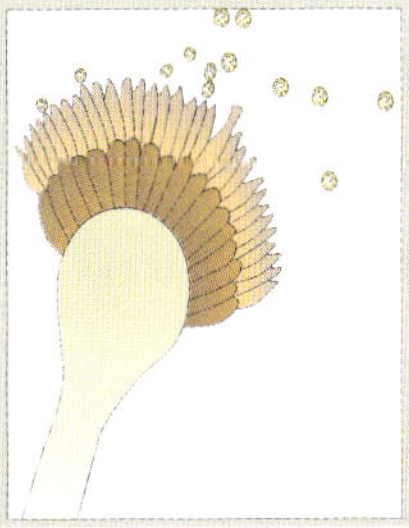

ASPERGILLUS FLAVUS

Macroscopic Morphology

- On Potato dextrose agar, colonies are granular, flat, often with radial grooves, yellow at first but quickly becoming bright to dark yellow-green with age (Fig. 8.5).

Microscopic Morphology

- Conidial heads are typically radiate, mostly 300-400 μm in diameter, later splitting to form loose columns, biseriate but having some heads with phialides borne directly on the vesicle. Conidiophores are hyaline and coarsely roughened, the roughness often being more noticeable near the vesicle (Fig. 8.6).
- Conidia are globose to subglobose (3-6 μm in diameter), pale green and conspicuously echinulate. Some strains produce brownish sclerotia.

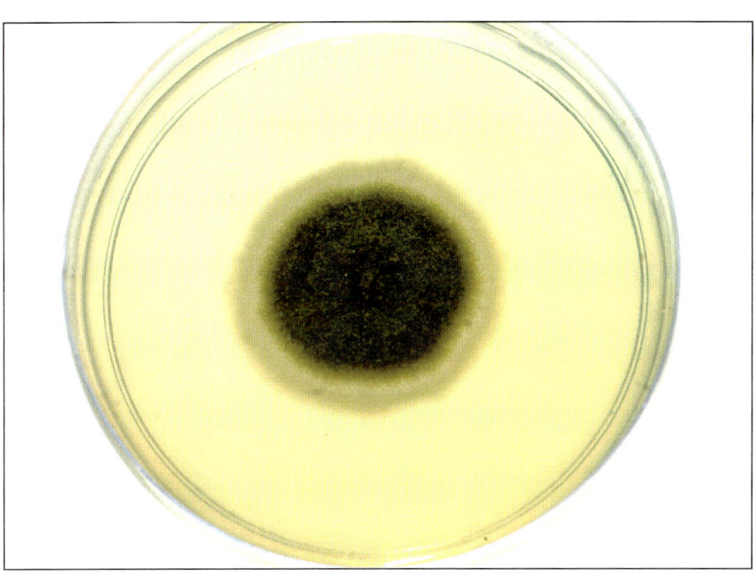

Fig. 8.5: *Aspergillus flavus* growth on potato dextrose agar, 25°C, 5 days

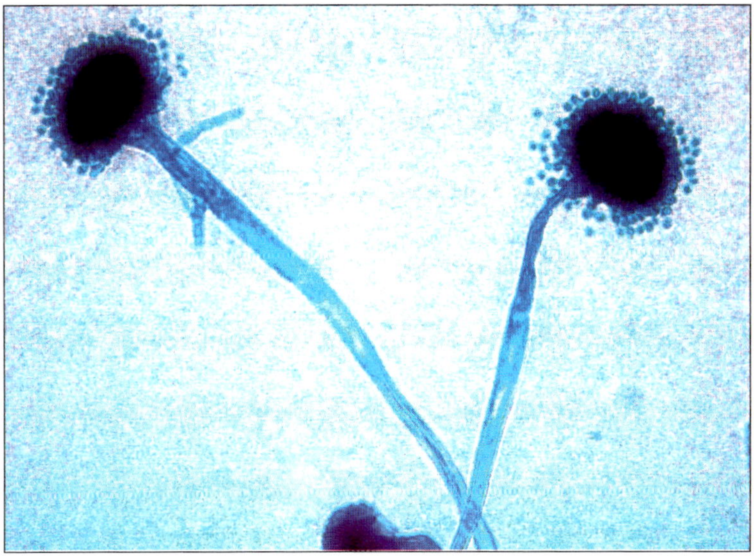

Fig. 8.6: *Aspergillus flavus* conidial head supported by a rough-walled conidiophore

ASPERGILLUS FUMIGATUS

Macroscopic Morphology

- On potato dextrose agar, colonies show typical blue-green surface pigmentation with a suede-like surface consisting of a dense felt of conidiophores (Figs 8.7A and B).

Microscopic Morphology

- Conidial heads are typically columnar (up to 400 × 50 μm but often much shorter and smaller) and uniseriate. Conidiophores are short, smooth-walled and have conical-shaped terminal vesicles which support a single row of phialides on the upper two thirds of the vesicle (Fig. 8.8). Conidia are produced in basipetal succession forming long chains and are globose to subglobose (2.5-3.0 μm in diameter), green and rough-walled.
- Note, this species is thermotolerant and grows at temperatures up to 55°C.

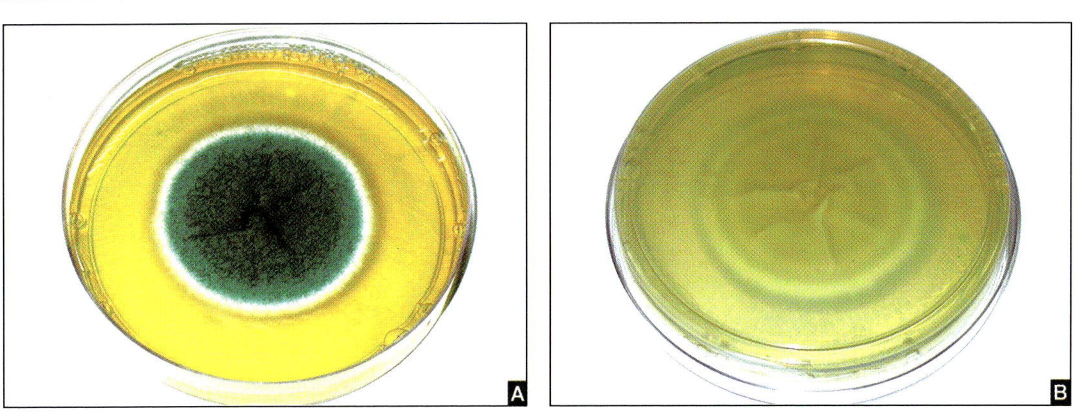

Figs 8.7A and B: *Aspergillus fumigatus* growth on Potato dextrose agar, 25°C, 5 days (A—Surface; B—Reverse)

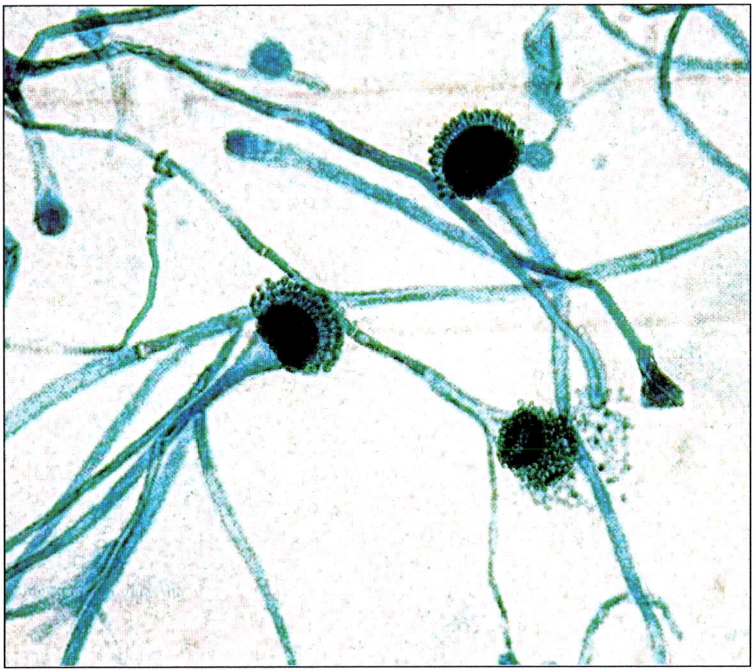

Fig. 8.8: *Aspergillus fumigatus* uniseriate phialides attached to the upper surface of the vesicle

ASPERGILLUS NIGER

Macroscopic Morphology

- On potato dextrose agar, colonies consist of a compact white or yellow basal felt covered by a dense layer of dark-brown to black conidial heads (Figs 8.9A and B).

Microscopic Morphology

- Conidial heads are large (up to 3 mm × 15-20 μm in diameter), globose, dark brown, becoming radiate and tending to split into several loose columns with age (Fig. 8.10).
- Conidiophores are smooth-walled, hyaline or turning dark towards the vesicle. Conidial heads are biseriate with the phialides borne on brown, often septate metulae.
- Conidia are globose to subglobose (3.5-5.0 μm in diameter), dark brown to black and rough-walled.

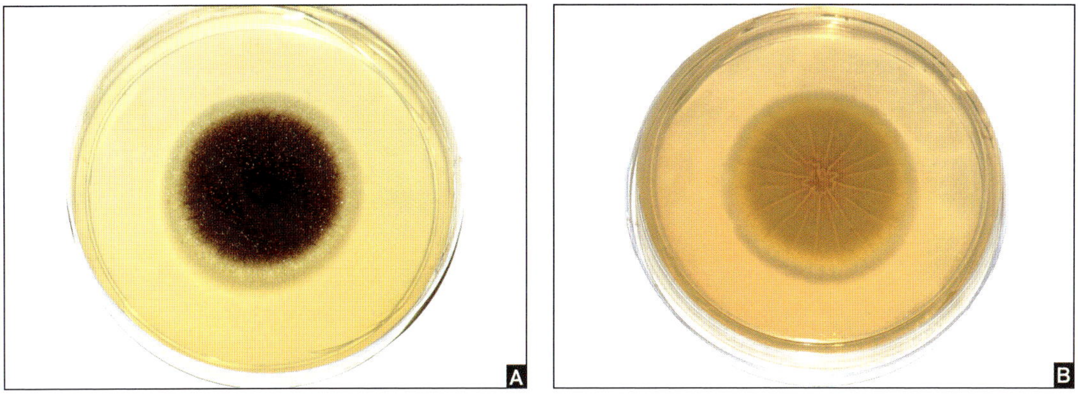

Figs 8.9A and B: *Aspergillus niger* growth on potato dextrose agar, 25°C, 5 days (**A**—Surface; **B**—Reverse)

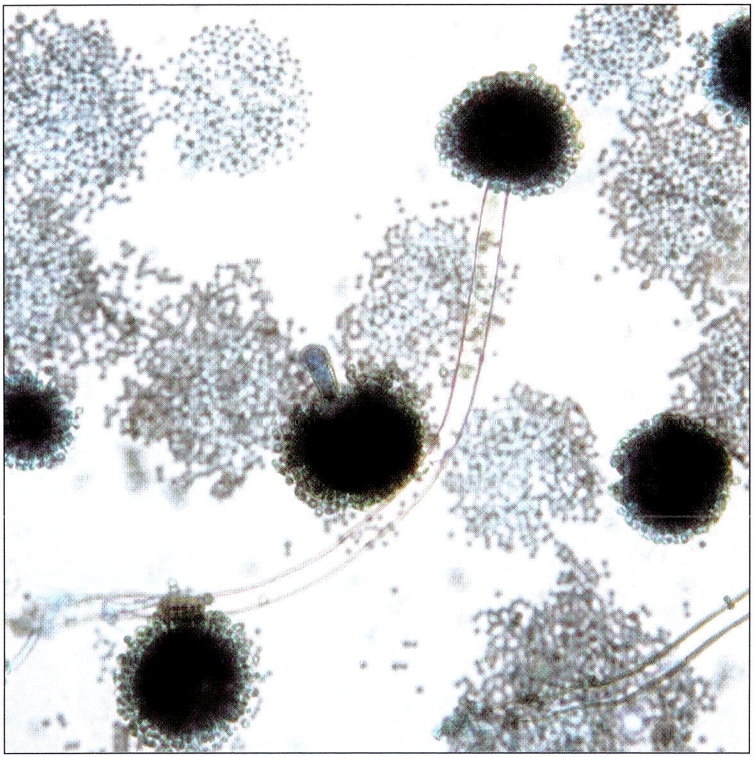

Fig. 8.10: *Aspergillus niger* with radiate conidial heads

ASPERGILLUS TERREUS

Macroscopic Morphology

- On potato dextrose agar, colonies are typically suede-like and cinnamon-buff to sand brown in color with a yellow to deep dirty brown reverse (Figs 8.11A and B).

Microscopic Morphology

- Conidial heads are compact, columnar (up to 500 × 30-50 μm in diameter) and biseriate (Figs 8.12A and B).
- Conidiophores are hyaline and smooth-walled.
- Conidia are globose to ellipsoidal (1.5-2.5 μm in diameter), hyaline to slightly yellow and smooth-walled.

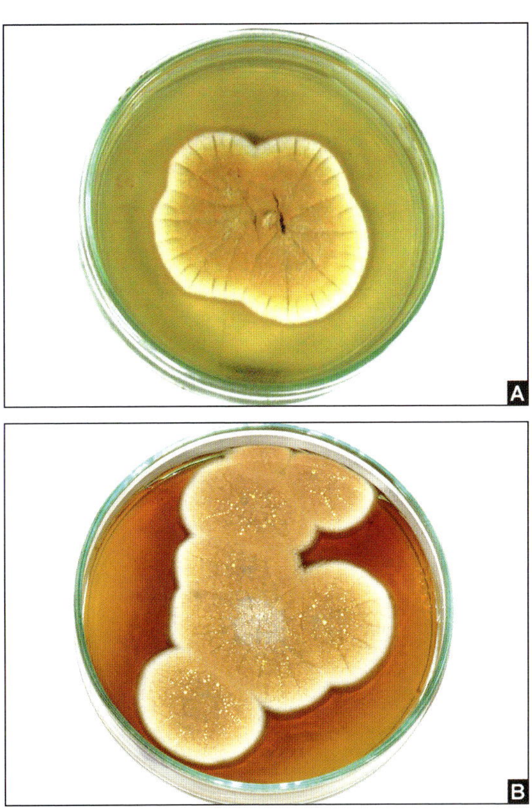

Figs 8.11A and B: *Aspergillus terreus* growth on potato dextrose agar, 25°C, 5 days (**A**—Pale cinnamon color coloy; **B**—Dark brown color colony)

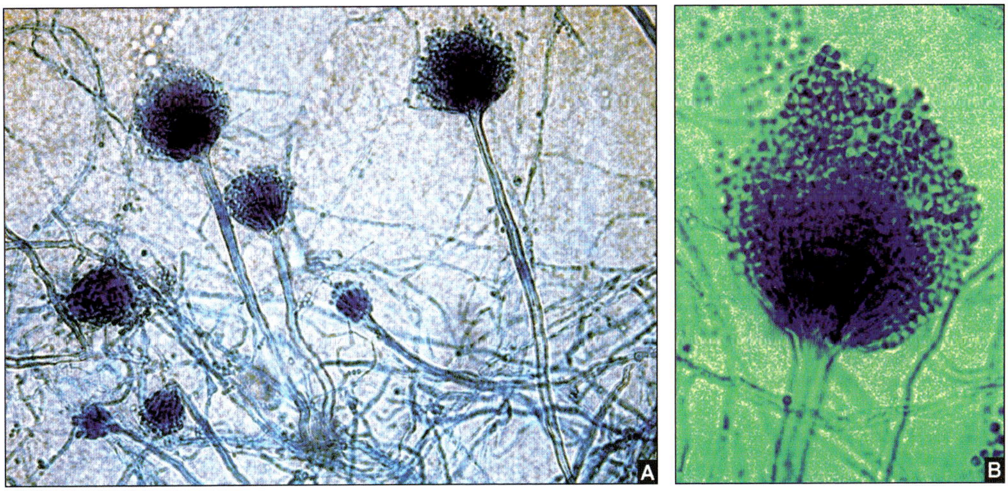

Figs 8.12A and B: *Aspergillus terreus* with biseriate conidial head

ASPERGILLUS NIDULANS

Macroscopic Morphology

On potato dextrose agar, colonies are typically pine green in color with tan to dark red-brown cleistothecia developing within and upon the conidial layer (Figs 8.13A and B). Reverse may be olive to drab-gray or purple-brown. Growth rate is slow to moderate in comparison with other clinically significant *Aspergillus* species.

Microscopic Morphology

- Conidial heads are short, columnar (up to 70 × 30 µm in diameter) and biseriate (Fig. 8.14).
- Conidiophores are usually short, brownish and smooth-walled.
- Vesicles are hemispherical, small (8-12 µm in diameter), with metulae and phialides occurring on the upper portion.
- Conidia are globose (3.0-3.5 µm in diameter) and rough-walled.
- *Aspergillus nidulans* is a homothallic species capable of producing the teleomorph (sexual stage) without mating studies. The ascomycetous telemorph *(Emericella nidulans)* produces brown to black globose cleistothecia (100-250 µm) that are surrounded with globose Hülle cells. Ascospores are reddish brown, lenticular (4 × 5 µm), with two equatorial crests.

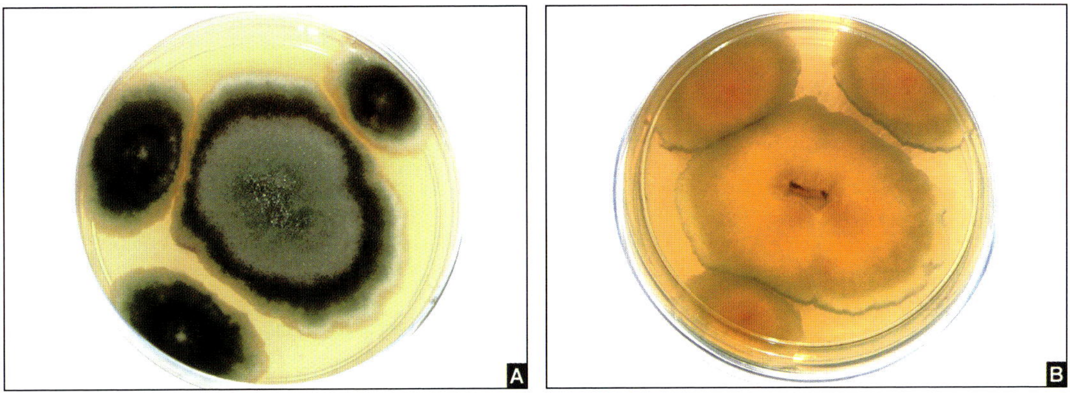

Figs 8.13A and B: *Aspergillus nidulans* growth on potato dextrose agar, 25°C, 7 days (**A**—Surface and **B**—Reverse)

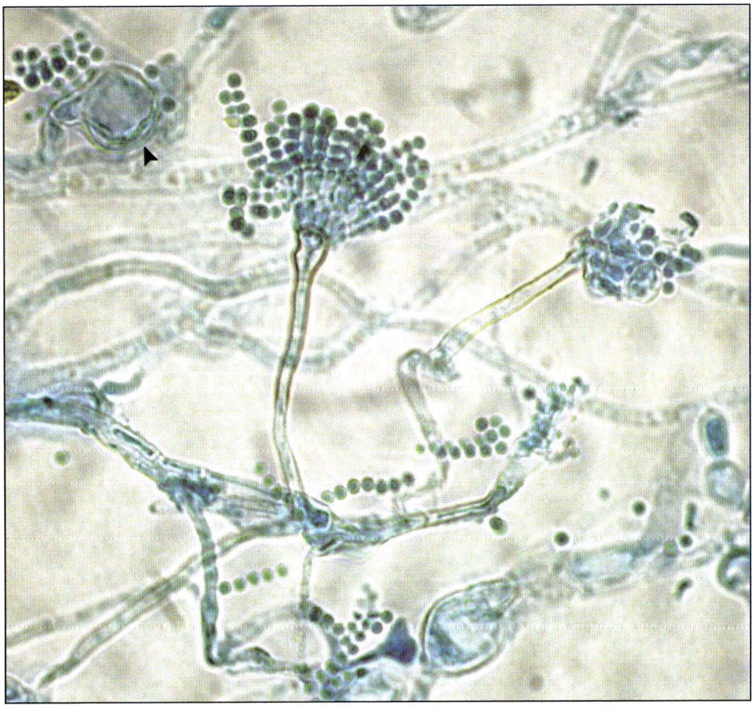

Fig. 8.14: *Aspergillus nidulans* conidial head and round hulle cells (➢)

ASPERGILLUS TAMARII

Ecology

A. tamarii is a member of *Aspergillus* section *Flavi*. Thisspecies is widely used in the food industry for the production of soy sauce (known as red Awamori koji) (14) and in the fermentation industry for the production of various enzymes, including amylases, proteases, and xylanolytic enzymes.

Pathogenicity

A. tamarii is able to produce several toxic secondary metabolites, including cyclopiazonic acid and fumigaclavines, it has rarely been encountered as a human pathogen. The only known cases are an eyelid infection, invasive nasosinusal aspergillosis in an immunocompetent patient, and onychomycosis in a 3-year-old boy.

The first cases of *A. tamarii fungal* keratitis reported by Kredics L et al, 2007 in Coimbatore, South India and they reported as fourth known case worldwide involving this unusual opportunistic human pathogen.

Macroscopic Morphology

- Colonies on malt extract agar at room temperature attained diameters of 6.0 to 7.0 cm in 10 days, producing abundant conidial heads in dull yellowish green shades becoming metallic bronze at maturity (Fig. 8.15).
- These are similar to *A. flavus* so their molecular identification only to differentate the species level.

Molecular Identification

DNA extraction:
- Masterpure yeast DNA purification kit (Epicenter Biotechnologies, Madison, WI).

DNA amplification:
- Primers 5.8S rRNA gene- ITS 1 and ITS 4
- Primers β-tubulin gene - bT2a and bTsb.

DNA sequencing:
- BigDye Terminator v3.1 cycle sequencing kit (Applied Biosystems Inc., foster city CA)
- ABI 3100 DNA Sequencer.

Microscopic Morphology

- The conidiophore stipe was hyaline and rough walled; the conidial heads were radiate; the vesicles were globose to subglobose, 25 to 50 μm in diameter.
- The phialides were borne directly on the vesicle or on metulae (mostly on large heads).
- The conidia were globose to subglobose, 5 to 6.5 μm in diameter, and brownish yellow. However, in contrast with those of typical wild *A. tamarii* isolates, some conidia of this isolate were not ornamented with tubercules and warts but were smooth walled and hyaline (Fig. 8.16).
- The isolate grew well at 37°C but was unable to grow at 42°C on malt extract agar medium.

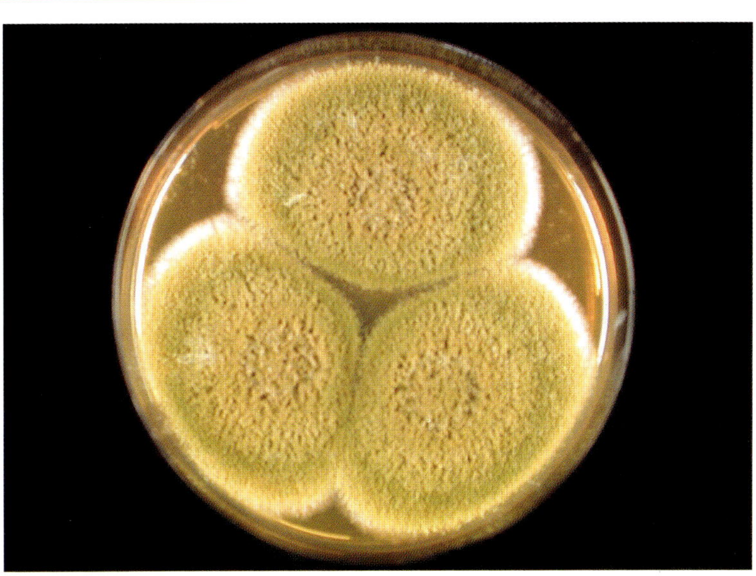

Fig. 8.15: Colony of *A.tamarii*

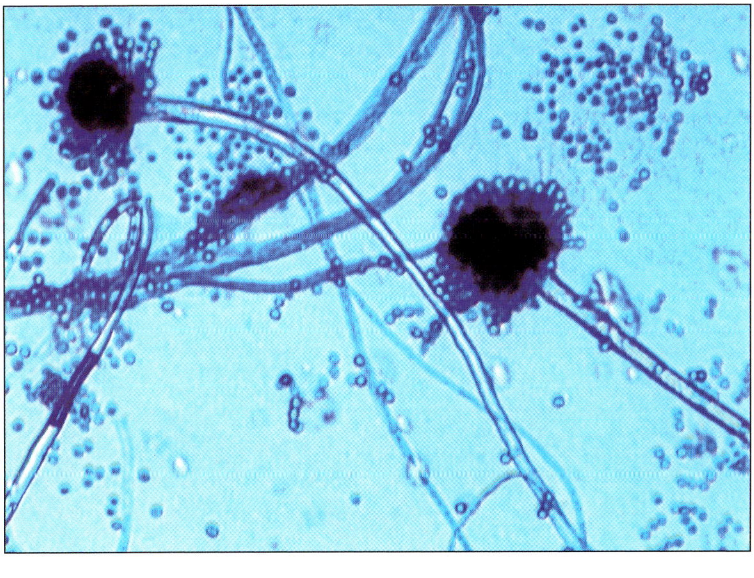

Fig. 8.16: Conidial head of *A. tamarii*

BIPOLARIS

Pathogenicity

Bipolaris is common cause of keratitis and endophthalmitis. Also occasionally the cause of diverse types of phaeohyphomycosis, including sinusitis, peritonitis, endocarditis, osteomyelitis, meningoencephalitis and cutaneous infection; these infections have been recognized in the immunocompromised patient as well as in the normal host.

Ecology

Cosmopolitan, although some species are mainly found in tropical or subtropical areas. Saprobes or pathogens of numerous species of plants.

Macroscopic Morphology

- *Bipolaris* colonies grow rapidly, reaching a diameter of 3 to 9 cm following incubation at 25°C for 7 days on potato dextrose agar (Figs 8.17A and B).
- The colony becomes mature within 5 days. The texture is velvety to woolly.
- The surface of the colony is initially white to grayish brown and becomes olive green to black with a raised grayish periphery as it matures.
- The reverse is also darkly pigmented and olive to black in color.

Microscopic Morphology

- The hyphae are septate and brown. Conidiophores (4.5-6 µm wide) are brown, simple or branched, geniculate or sympodial, bending at the points where each conidium arises.
- This property leads to the zigzag appearance of the conidiophore. The conidia, which are also called poroconidia, are 3- to 6-celled, fusoid to cylindrical in shape, light to dark brown in color and have sympodial geniculate growth pattern. The poroconidium (30-35 µm × 11-13.5 µm) is distoseptate and has a scarcely protuberant, darkly pigmented hilum (Fig. 8.18).
- This basal scar indicates the point of attachment to the conidiophore. From the terminal cell of the conidium, germ tubes may develop and elongate in the direction of longitudinal axis of the conidium.
- Teleomorph production of *Bipolaris* is heterothallic. The perithecium is black in color, and round to ellipsoidal in shape. The ascospores are flagelliform or filiform, hyaline in nature and are found in clavate-shaped or cylindrical asci. Each ascus contains eight ascospores.

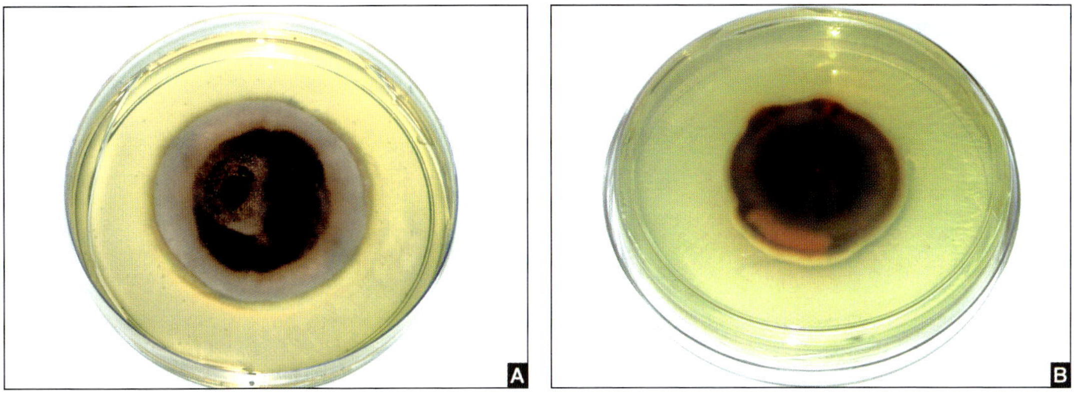

Figs 8.17A and B: *Bipolaris* species growth on potato dextrose agar, 25°C, 5 days (**A**—Surface; **B**—Reverse)

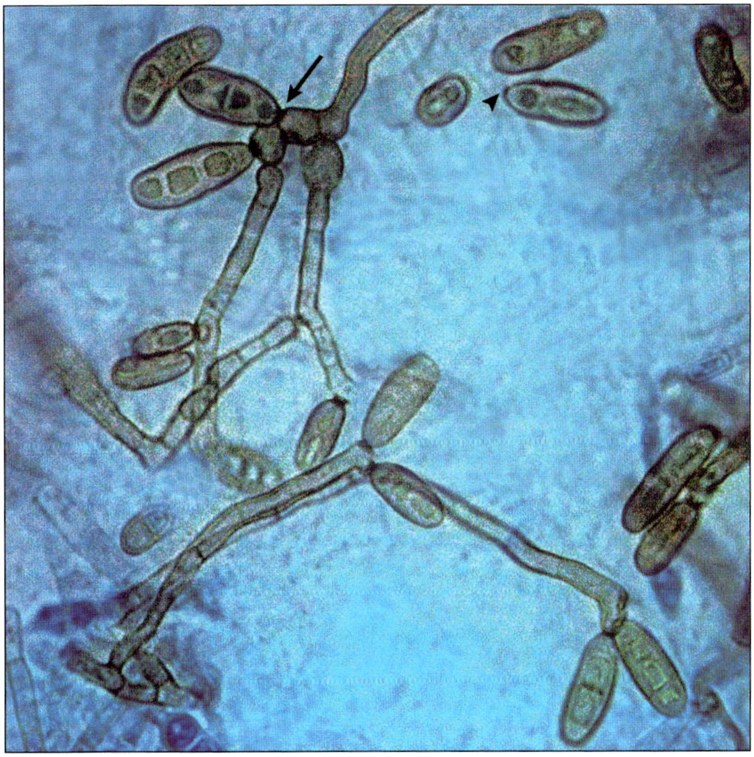

Fig. 8.18: *Bipolaris* species conidiophore geniculate with fusoid multiseptate conidia (→) scarcely protuberant hilum (➢)

CANDIDA

Ecology

Candida is a genus of yeasts. Clinically, the most significant member of the genus is *Candida albicans*, which can cause numerous infections (called candidiasis or thrush) in humans and other animals, especially in immunocompromised patients. (Ryan KJ et al, 2004). Various *Candida* species are members of gut flora in animals, including *C. albicans*.

Pathogenicity

C. albicans is the most common cause of both superficial and systemic candidosis. It is also often present as part of the commensal flora of the mouth, vaginal mucosa and gastrointestinal tract, and may be isolated from these sites in the absence of disease.

Most episodes of yeast infections in corneal ulcers and other ocular infections are due to various *Candida* species, predominantly *Candida albicans* and usually occur in the presence of systemic illness (diabetes mellitus or immunocompromise) or ocular diseases like lid abnormalities or dry eyes) or endogenous endophthalmitis and in patients receiving prolonged topical medications or topical corticosteroids.

Macroscopic Morphology

- *Candida albicans* grows well on potato dextrose agar (Fig. 8.19), Sabouraud's agar and most routinely used bacteriological media.
- Convex, entire margin, non-mucoid, smooth texture of cream colored pasty colonies usually appear after 24 - 48 hours incubation at 35-37°C.
- The colonies have a distinctive yeast smell.

Microscopic Morphology

- The round—oval shaped budding cells can be easily seen by direct microscopy in stained or unstained preparations.
- *Candida albicans* produces true germ tubes when incubated in serum for 2-3 hours at 37°C (Fig. 8.20).
- These are parallel-sided tubes which are formed at right angles to the parent cell and are at least twice as long as the parent cell before cross walls are formed.

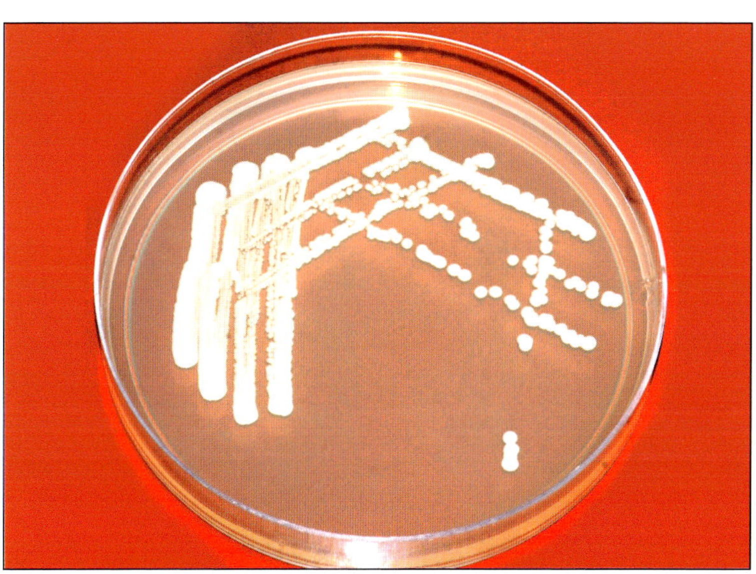

Fig. 8.19: Cream colored pasty colonies on potato dextrose agar (2 days)

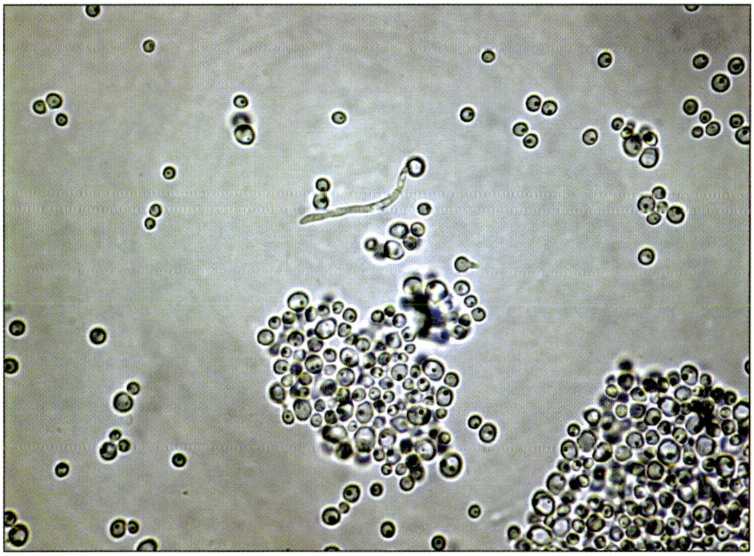

Fig. 8.20: *C.albicans* produces true germ tubes

CEPHALIOPHORA IRREGULARIS

Ecology

The genus cephaliophora contains coprophilous fungi. In India, they are generally found growing on the dung of rats. They have also been reported from moist wood. There are two species known to be prevalent in India: *Cephaliophora tropica* and *Cephaliophora irregularis.* The genus *Cephaliophora* was established by Thaxter in 1903 as a new genus of Deuteromycetes consists of two species of dung inhabiting fungi. One species, *C.irregularis* Thaxter was isolated from mouse dung. *C.tropica* was isolated from the dung of various animals from Jamaica, Liberia, Java and China.

Pathogenicity

In 1990 Thomas et al reported a first case of human infection of keratitis caused by *C. irregularis* from Tiruchirapalli, South India. The second case of mycotic keratitis due to *C.irregularis* reported from Christian Medical College, Vellore (Mathews 1995).

Macroscopic Morphology (Fig. 8.21)

- Rapid growth
- Hyaline mycelial growth
- Later became cottony without a pigment being formed
- Colonies on blood agar had a similar appearance.

Microscopic Morphology (Figs 8.22A to C)

- Revealed hyaline, short, sessile, septate and solitary conidiophores
- Bearing clusters of pale brown conidia
- The conidia were mostly two-celled, pyriform or triangular.

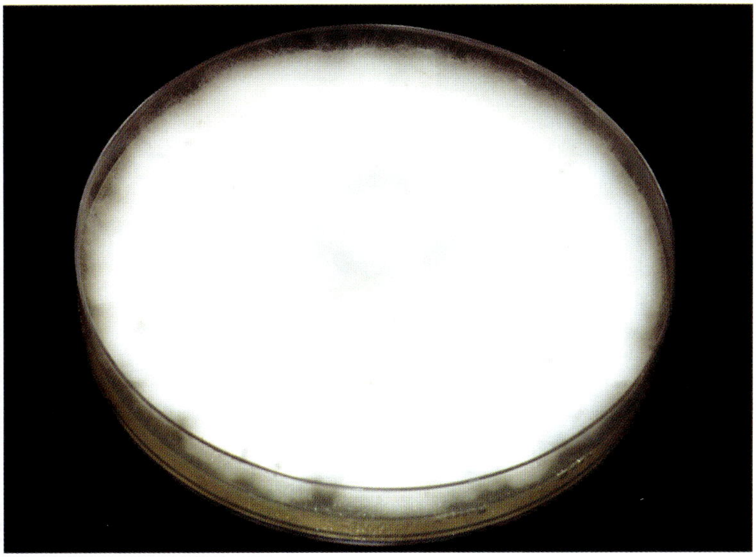

Fig. 8.21: Cottony white colony of *C.irregularis* on potato dextrose agar (7 days)

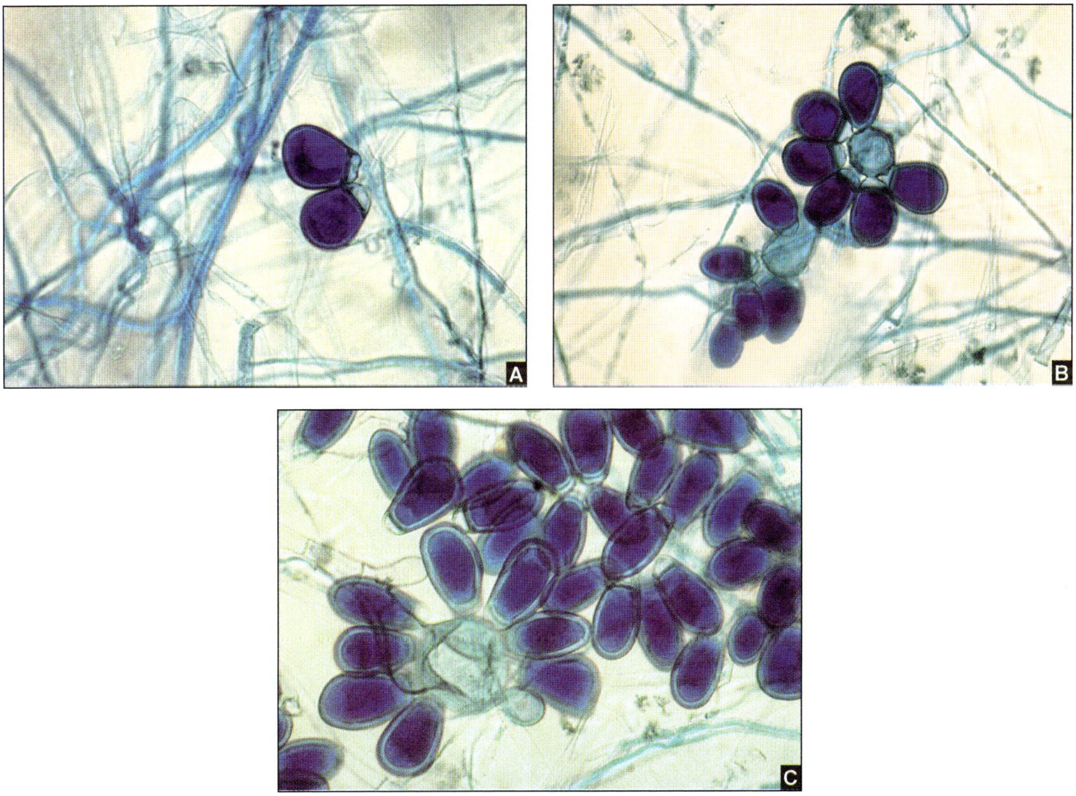

Figs 8.22A to C: Two conidium (**A**) and Cluster of conidia borne on short swollen conidiogenous cells **B** and **C** (400 X magnification)

CLADOSPORIUM

Pathogenicity

One of the most common dematiaceous fungi to cause keratitis and endophthalmitis. Generally nonpathogenic, with the exception of *Cladosporium carrionii* an agent of chromoblastomycosis. This is a chronic subcutaneous infection characterized by verrucous lesion and the formation of brown, sclerotic fission cells (copper pennies) in tissue. It is often confined to a single limb.

Ecology

Many species are cosmopolitan fungi or soil, plant debris and leaf surfaces. *Cladosporium* is very frequently isolated from air, especially during seasons in which humidity is elevated.

Macroscopic Morphology

- The growth rate of *Cladosporium* colonies is moderate on potato dextrose agar at 25°C and the texture is velvety to powdery (Figs 8.23A and B). Similar to the other dematiaceous fungi, the color is olivaceous green to black from the front and black from the reverse.
- Most of the *Cladosporium* spp. do not grow at temperatures above 35°C.

Microscopic Morphology

- *Cladosporium* spp. produces septate brown hyphae, erect and pigmented conidiophores, and conidia.
- Conidia of *Cladosporium* spp. in general are elliptical to cylindrical in shape, pale to dark brown in color and have dark hila (Fig. 8.24). They occur in branching chains that readily disarticulate. Conidial wall is smooth or occasionally echinulate.

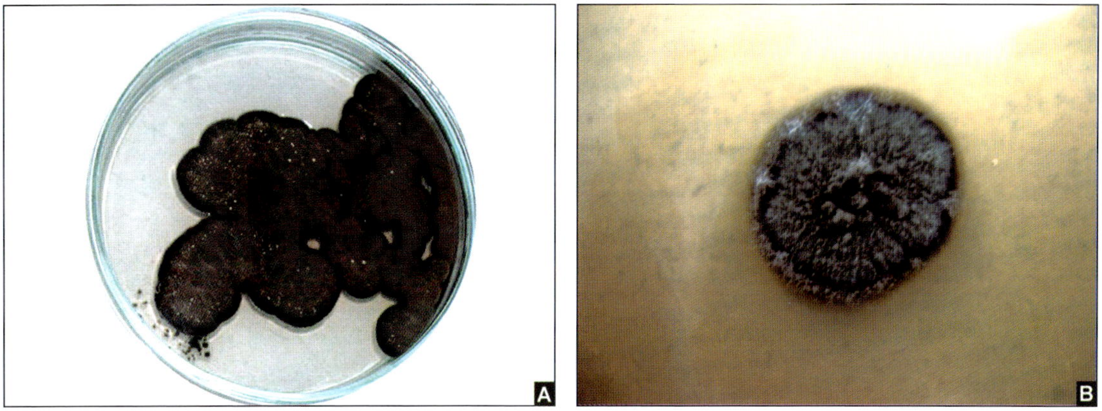

Figs 8.23A and B: *Cladosporium* species growth on potato dextrose agar, 25°C, 5 days

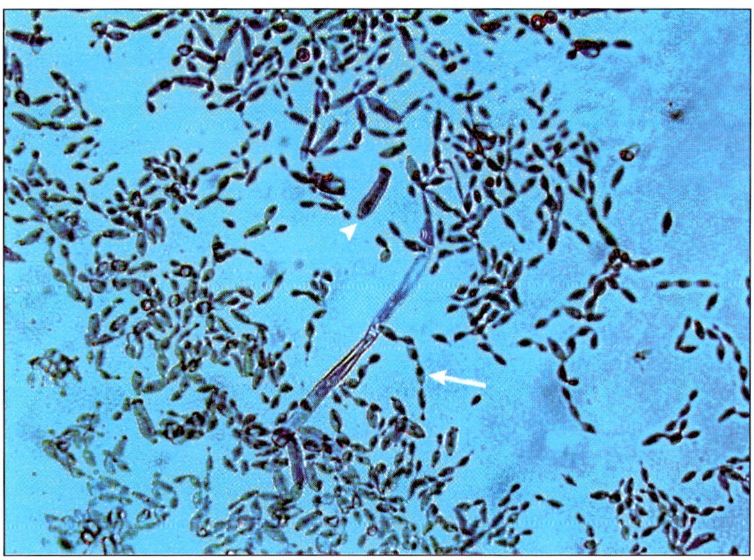

Fig. 8.24: *Cladosporium* species Shield-shaped conidia with scars (➢) at points of attachment, bicellular conidium (→)

COLLETOTRICHUM SPP

Pathogenicity

Colletotrichum generally associated with some form of trauma. They manifest as keratitis or subcutaneous lesions, although a case of invasive infections has been reported. Five species of *Colletotrichum* have been reported to cause infections in humans. They are *Colletotrichum coccodes, C.crassipes, C. dematium, C. gloeosporioides,* and *C. graminicola*. The predominant infection is keratitis following traumatic implantation, but subcutaneous and systemic infections among immunosuppressed patients have also been reported.

Ecology

The genus *Colletotrichum* is one of the most important genera of plant pathogens. It has a worldwide distribution but is found mainly in subtropical and tropical regions. *Colletotrichum* species cause economically significant diseases of plants (generally referred to as anthracnoses) that affect cereals and grasses, legumes, vegetables, and perennial crops, including fruit trees.

Macroscopic Morphology (Figs 8.25, 8.26A and B)

Colonies usually darkly pigmented with white aerial mycelium, consisting of numerous black sclerotia and light brown colored conidial masses, reverse is dark brown.

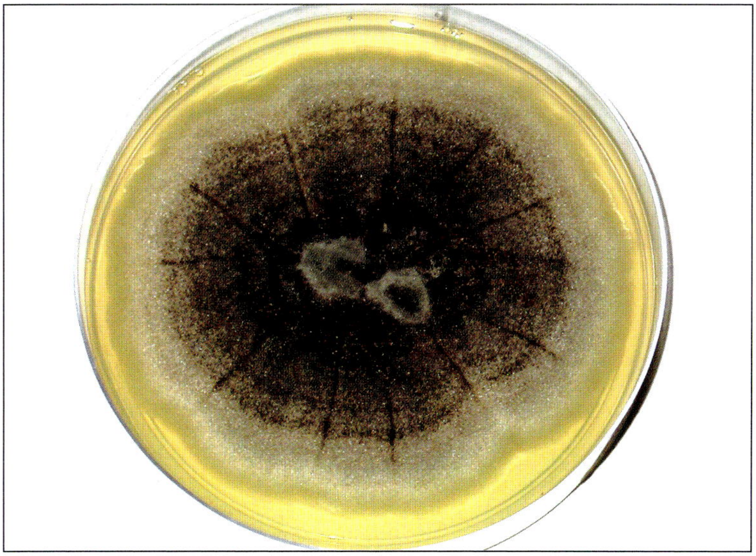

Fig. 8.25: *Colletotrichum* species growth on potato dextrose agar, 25°C, 7days

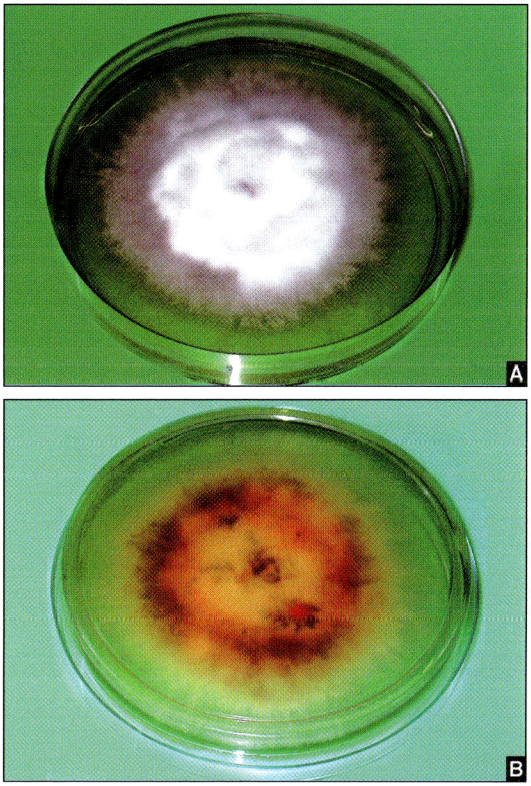

Figs 8.26A and B: 5 days old culture of *C. coccodes* (**A**—Surface; **B**—Reverse)

Microscopic Morphology (Figs 8.27 and 8.28)

- Sclerotia are usually abundant, setose, spherical and are often confluent.
- Conidia are straight, fusiform, attenuated at the ends, 16-22 × 3-4 μm. Appressoria are common, clavate, brown, 11-16.5 × 6-9.5 μm.
- The key morphological features which identify the genus are its acervular conidiomata, often with ***setae*** (dark-pigmented, unbranched, thick-walled sterile hyphae usually pointed at the tip), producing elongated slimy conidia, and the presence of appressoria (thick-walled swellings at the end of a hypha or germ tube useful for attaching the fungus to the host surface before penetration of the tissue).

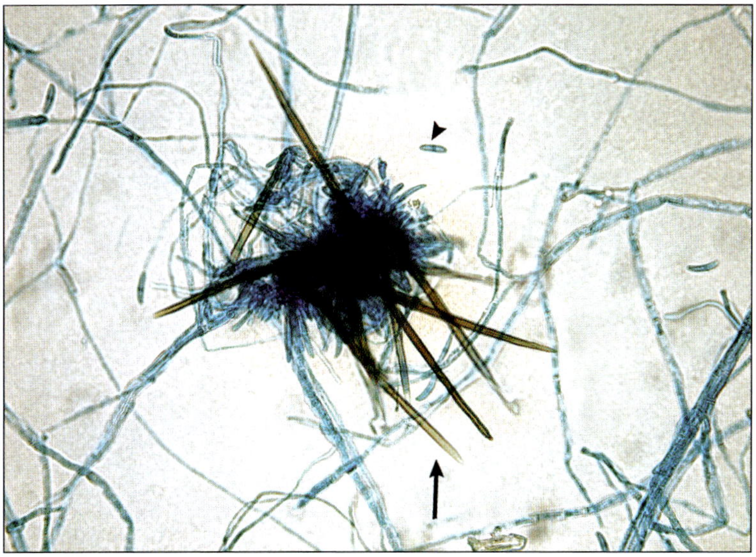

Fig. 8.27: Few conidia (➤) with setae (→) of *Colletotrichum*

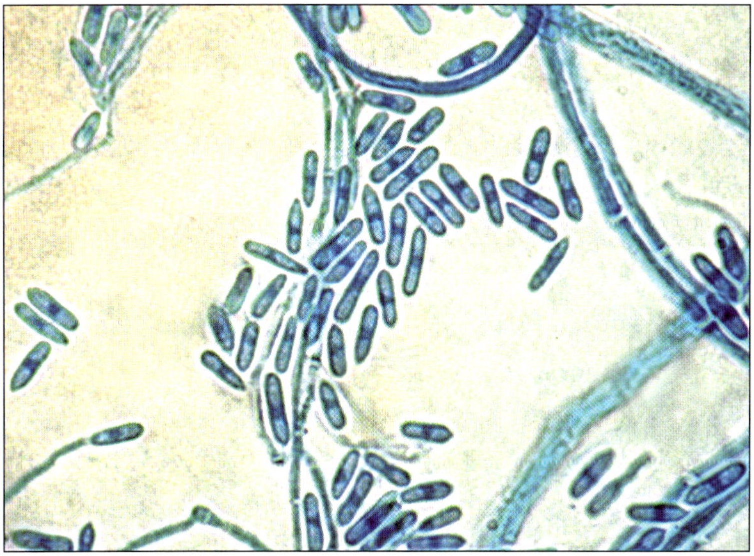

Fig. 8.28: Cylindrical conidia of *Colletotrichum coccodes*

CURVULARIA

Pathogenicity

Infection of the cornea, reported in 1959, was the first human disease proved to be caused by *Curvularia*. It is the most common dematiaceous fungus to cause corneal ulcer. Other ocular infections consist of conjunctivitis, dacryocytitis, sino-orbital cellulites, and endophthalmitis. But the cornea is the most commonly infected site.

Several *Curvularia* species are zoo pathogenic. Wound infection is the most common disease caused by *Curvularia* and ranges from onychomycosis to skin ulceration and subcutaneous mycetoma. Other human *Curvularia* infections are invasive and allergic sinusitis and bronchopulmonary disease. Abscesses of the lung, brain, liver, and connective tissue have occurred. Nosocomial infections include dialysis-related peritonitis and post surgical endocarditis.

Ecology

Most species are facultative pathogens of tropical or subtropical plants, but a few are commonly isolated in temperate agricultural areas.

Macroscopic Morphology (Fig. 8.29)

- *Curvularia* produces rapidly growing, woolly colonies on potato dextrose agar at 25°C.
- From the front, the color of the colony is white to pinkish gray initially and turns to olive brown or black as the colony matures.
- From the reverse, it is dark brown to black.

Microscopic Morphology

- Septate, brown hyphae, brown conidiophores, and conidia are visualized. Conidiophores are simple or branched and are bent at the points where the conidia originate. This bending pattern is called sympodial geniculate growth.
- The conidia (8-14 × 21-35 µm), which are also called the poroconidia, are straight to pyriform, brown, multiseptate, and have dark basal protuberant hila (Fig. 8.30).
- The septa are transverse and divide each conidium into multiple cells. The central cell is typically darker and enlarged compared to the end cells in the conidium.
- The central septum may also appear darker than the others. The swelling of the central cell usually gives the conidium a curved appearance.
- The number of the septa, shape (straight or curved),color of the conidia (dark vs pale brown), as well as the existence of dark median septum, and the prominence of geniculate growth pattern are the major microscopic features that help in differentiation of *Curvularia* spp. among each other.
- For instance, the conidia of *Curvularia lunata* have 3 septa and 4 cells, while those of *Curvularia geniculata* mostly have 4 septa and 5 cells.

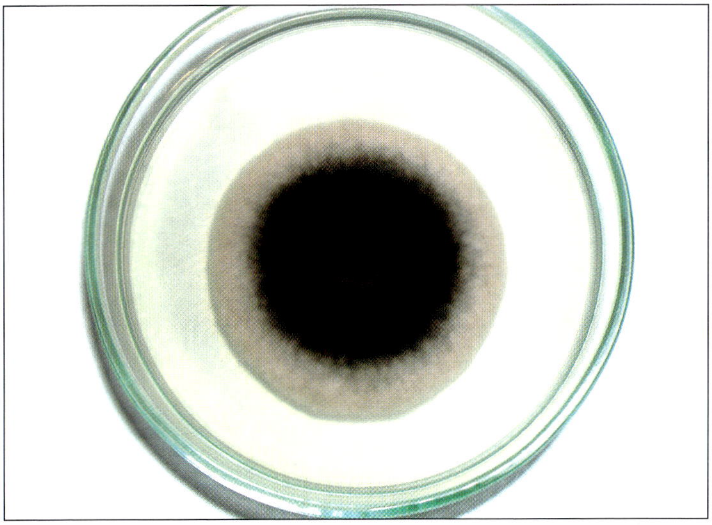

Fig. 8.29: *Curvularia* species growth on Potato dextrose agar, 25°C, 5 days

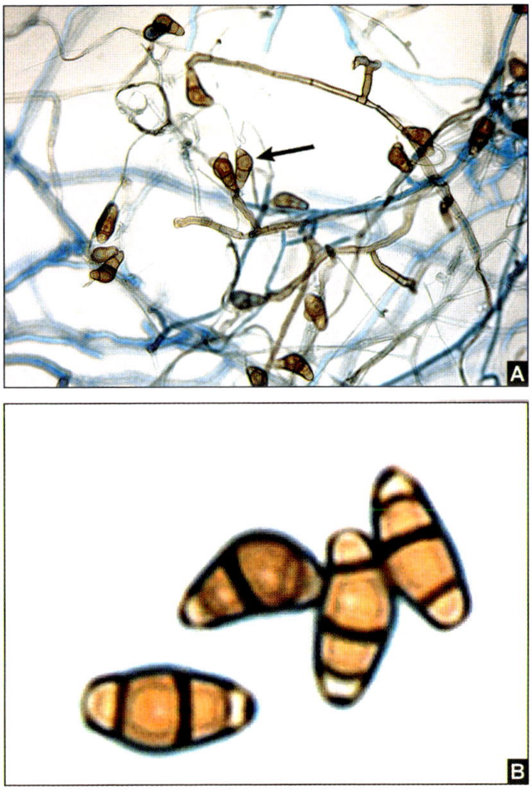

Figs 8.30A and B: *Curvularia* species growth curved poroconidia with larger and darker central cell (→)

EXSEROHILUM

Pathogenicity

One of the common dematiaceous fungus to cause keratitis.

Exserohilum species cause phaehyphomycosis affecting skin, sub cutaneous tissue, nose and paranasal sinuses, rarely endocarditis and osteomyelitis. Some cases of subcutaneous or deep phaehyphomycosis have been reported in humans and animals.

Ecology

Cosmopolitan, facultative plant pathogens, also occasionally isolated from soil.

Macroscopic Morphology (Fig. 8.31)

- Moderately rapid growth
- Texture velvety
- Color dark olive to black on the surface and reverse.

Microscopic Morphology (Fig. 8.32)

- Hyphae septate, pale brown
- Conidiophores brown, geniculate at the apex
- Proconidia cylindrical to ellipsoidal, multicellular, distoseptate with a protuberant hilum at the base
- Germ tubes developing in the direction of the conidial long axis or on the side.

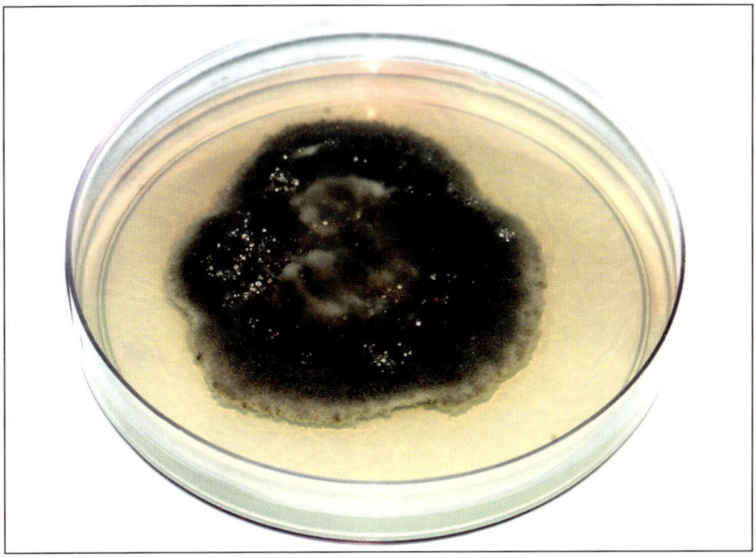

Fig. 8.31: *Exserohilum* species growth on potato dextrose agar, 25°C, 7 days

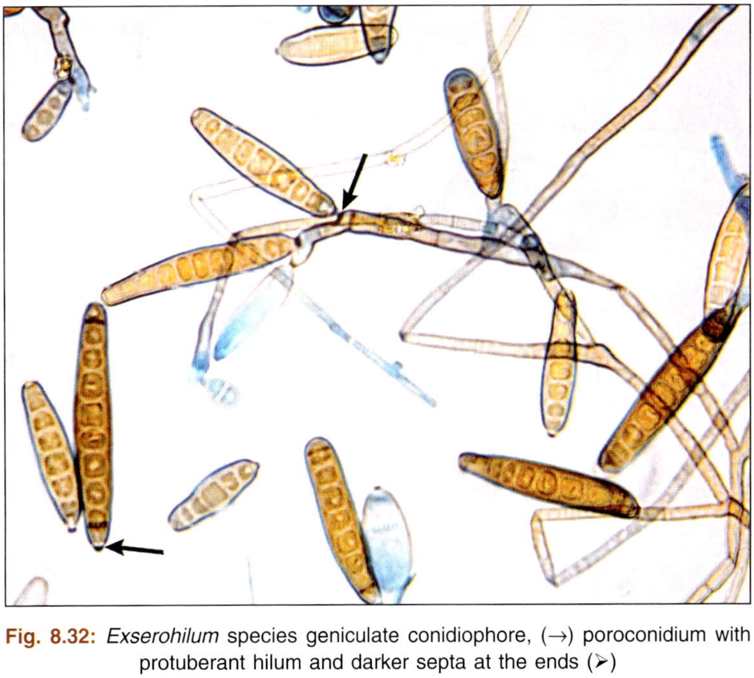

Fig. 8.32: *Exserohilum* species geniculate conidiophore, (→) poroconidium with protuberant hilum and darker septa at the ends (➢)

FUSARIUM

Pathogenicity

Species of Fusarium are widespread saprobic fungi that cause important diseases of plants, particularly major crop plants and of humans. They have long been regarded as important pathogens in eye infections, especially keratitis.

As well as being common plant pathogens, *Fusarium* spp are causative agents of superficial and systemic infections in humans. Infections due to *Fusarium* spp. are collectively referred to as fusariosis. The most virulent *Fusarium* spp is *Fusarium solani*. Trauma is the major predisposing factor for development of cutaneous infections due to *Fusarium* strains. Disseminated opportunistic infections, on the other hand, develop in immunosuppressed hosts, particularly in neutropenic and transplant patients. *Fusarium* infections following solid organ transplantation tend to remain local and have a better outcome compared to those that develop in patients with hematological malignancies and bone marrow transplantation patients.

Keratitis, endophthalmitis, otitis media, onychomycosis, cutaneous infections particularly of burn wounds, mycetoma, sinusitis, pulmonary infections, endocarditis, peritonitis, central venous catheter infections, septic arthritis, disseminated infections, and fungemia due to *Fusarium* spp. have been reported.

Outbreaks of nosocomial fusariosis have also been reported. Existence of *Fusarium* in hospital water distribution systems may result in disseminated fusariosis in immunosuppressed patients. *Fusarium* may also exist in soil of potted plants in hospitals. These plants constitute a hazardous mycotic reservoir for nosocomial fusariosis.

Clusters of *Fusarium* keratitis were reported among contact lens users in Asia beginning in February 2006.

Ecology

Cosmopolitan, frequently isolated from soil. Certain species are important plant pathogens, other produce toxins in grains or stored animal feed.

- *Fusarium solani*
- *F. oxysporum*
- *F. dimerum*.

Macroscopic Morphology (Figs 8.33 and 8.34)

- *Fusarium* spp. grow rapidly on Sabouraud's dextrose agar at 25°C and produce woolly to cottony, flat, spreading colonies. The only slow-growing species is *Fusarium dimerum* (Figs 8.35A and B).
- From the front, the color of the colony may be white, cream, tan, salmon, cinnamon, yellow, red, violet, pink, or purple. From the reverse, it may be colorless, tan, red, dark purple or brown.

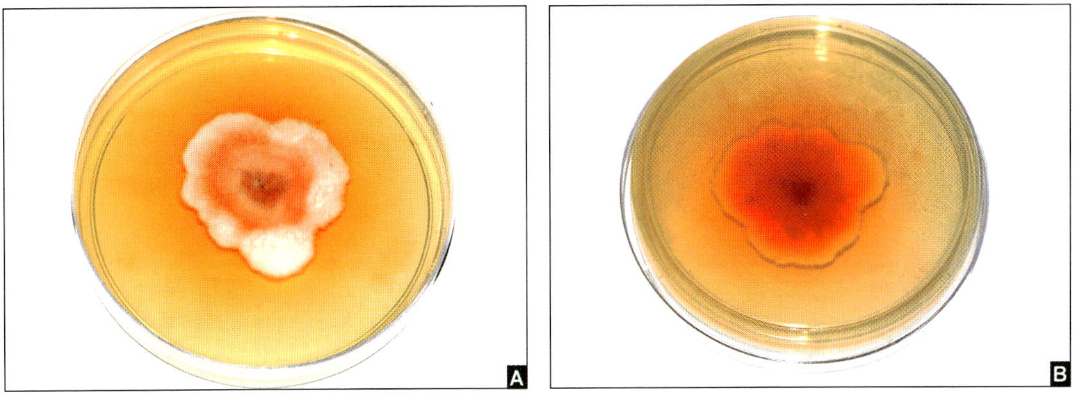

Figs 8.33A and B: *Fusarium* species growth on potato dextrose agar, 25°C, 5 days (**A**—Surface; **B**—Reverse)

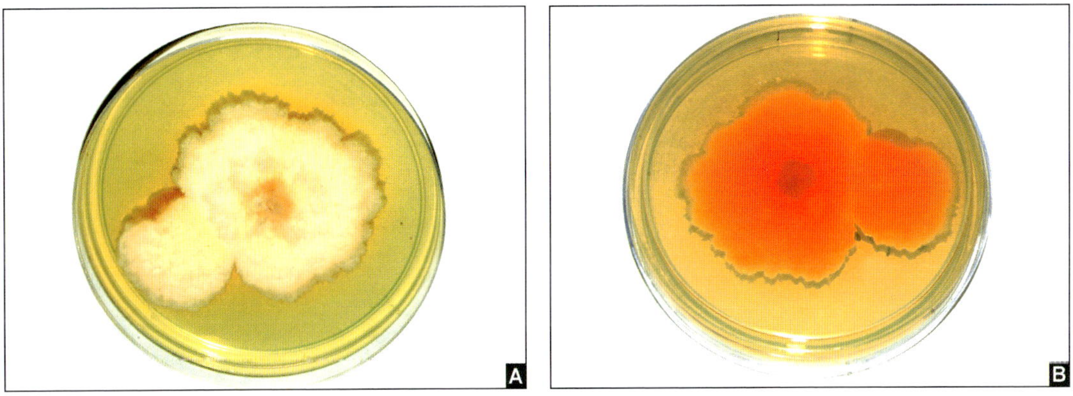

Figs 8.34A and B: *F. semitectum* (**A**—Surface; **B**—Reverse)

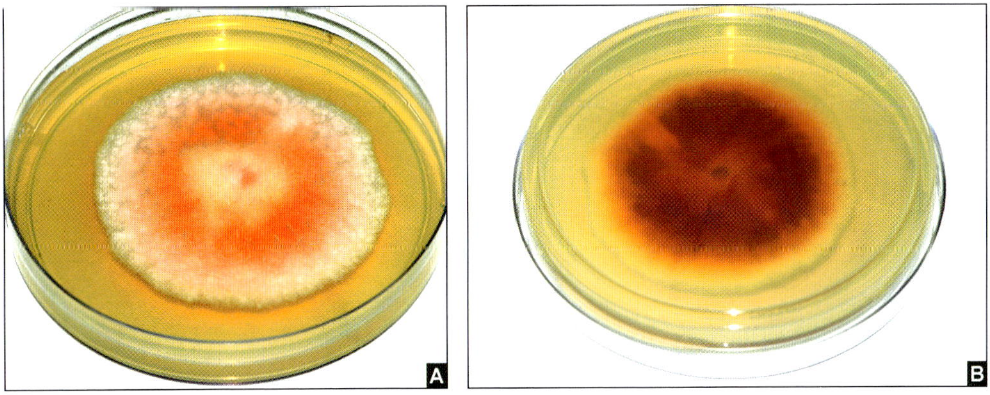

Figs 8.35A and B: *F. dimerum* (**A**—Surface; **B**—Reverse)

- A sclerotium, which is the organized mass of hyphae that remains dormant during unfavorable conditions, may be observed macroscopically and is usually dark blue in color.
- On the other hand the sporodochium a cushion-like, moist mat of hyphae bearing conidiophores over its surface, is usually absent in culture. When present, it may be observed in cream to tan or orange color, except for, which gives rise to blue-green or blue sporodochia.

Microscopic Morphology

- Hyaline septate hyphae, conidiophores, phialides, macroconidia, and microconidia are observed microscopically. In addition to these basic elements, chlamydospores are also produced by *Fusarium* chamydosporum, *Fusarium napiforme, Fusarium oxysporum, Fusarium solani* (Figs 8.36A and B), *Fusarium semitectum* (Fig. 8.37) *and Fusarium sporotrichoides.*
- Phialides are cylindrical, with a small collarette, solitary or produced as a component of a complex branching system. Monophialides and polyphialides (in heads or in chains) may be observed. Macroconidia (3-8 × 11-70 µm) are produced from phialides on unbranched or branched conidiophores. They are 2- or more celled, thick-walled, smooth, and cylindrical or sickle-shaped.
- Macroconidia have a distinct basal foot cell and pointed distal ends. They tend to accumulate in balls or rafts. Microconidia (2-4 × 4-8 µm), on the other hand, are formed on long or short simple conidiophores. They are 1-celled (occasionally 2- or 3-celled), smooth, hyaline, ovoid to cylindrical, and arranged in balls (occasionally occurring in chains).
- Chlamydospores sometimes present. They are thick-walled, hyaline, intercalary or terminal.
- Macroscopic and microscopic features, such as color of the colony; length and shape of the macroconidia, the number, shape and arrangement of microconidia, and presence or absence of chlamydospores are key features for the differentiation of *Fusarium* species.

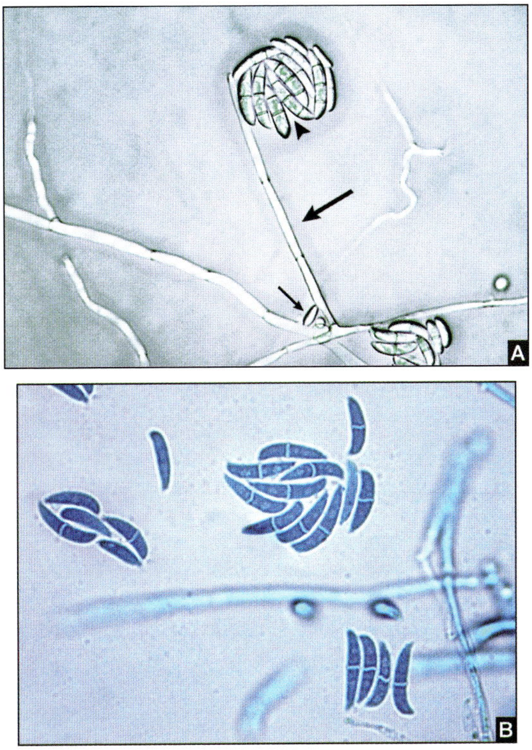

Figs 8.36A and B: Macroconidium with foot cell of *F. solani* (➢macroconidium; → microconidia; ⟶ foot cell)

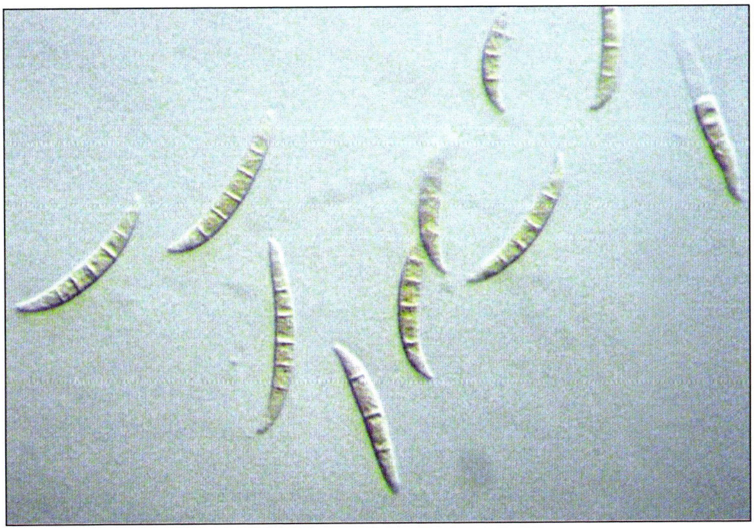

Fig. 8.37: Macroconidium of *F. semitectum*

LASIODIPLODIA THEOBROMAE

Ecology

Worldwide, well known plant pathogen.

Pathogenicity

Lasiodiplodia theobromae is a widespread saprophyte and wound-parasite on a considerable range of hosts in the tropics. It is an important parasite of bananas in storage, causing several forms of fruit-rot. *Lasiodiplodia theobromae,* a rare cause of mycotic keratitis and endophthalmitis.

Macroscopic Morphology

- Colonies on potato dextrose agar greyish sepia to mouse grey to black, fluffy with abundant aerial mycelium (Fig. 8.38).
- Colonies reverse fuscous black to black.

Microscopic Morphology (Fig. 8.39)

- Conidia initially unicellular, hyaline, granulose, subovoid to ellipsoide-oblong, thick-walled, base truncate; mature conidia 1-septate, cinnamon to fawn, often longitudinally striate, (18-) 20-30 × 10-15 µm.
- The pycnospores are elliptical, at first unicellular and hyaline, becoming brown and 1-septate, sometimes with longitudinal striations, 20-30 × 10-18 µm.

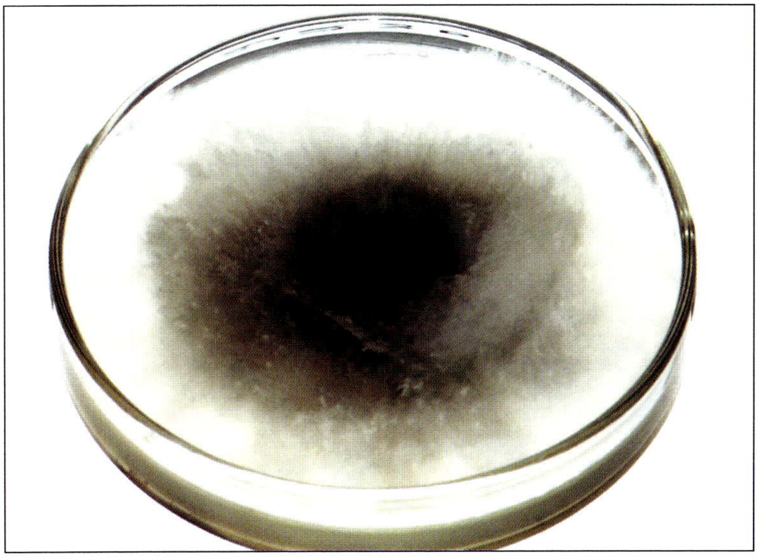

Fig. 8.38: *Lasiodiplodia theobromae* growth on potato dextrose agar (10 days)

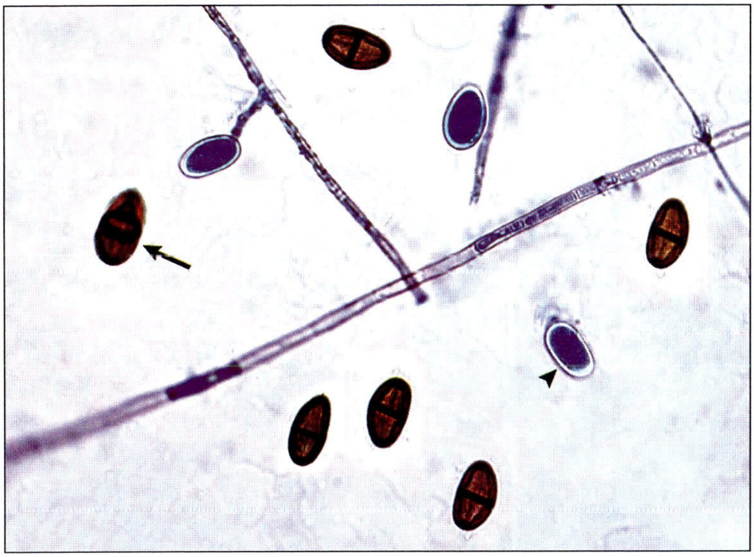

Fig. 8.39: Two-celled, pigmented pycnidioconidia of *L. theobromae*
(➢Young conidia; → Matured conidia)

NEOCOSMOSPORA VASINFECTA

Ecology

The genus *Neocosmospora* was established by Smith for a species apparently pathogenic to various crops including cotton, watermelon and cowpea in the southeastern United States. *Neocosmospora vasinfecta*, a filamentous ascomycete belonging to the Hypocreales order of the Ascomycota division is a common plant pathogen predominantly found in tropical and subtropical areas.

Pathogenicity

It has rarely been reported as being responsible for infections in humans. Known cases include a leg granuloma in a renal transplant recipient, post-traumatic osteoarthritis in an immunocompetent patient, a fatal disseminated infection in a patient with acute nonlymphocytic leukemia and an infection in a pediatric burn patient.

Occupational exposure to cotton may be a risk factor as *N. vasinfecta* has been isolated from intact senescent cotton roots. Although *N. vasinfecta* has been reported to occur in plants in India, according to our knowledge, human infections due to this fungus has not been previously described in this country. Due to their rarity, l-break/> *N. vasinfecta* infections are often treated as if caused by *Fusarium* species, because the cultural morphology.

Macroscopic Morphology

- Colonies of the fungus were fast growing on PDA at 25°C, flat, thin and appeared almost transparent at first with obvious rings forming as the colonies matured (Fig. 8.40).
- In early stage colonies are very similar to *Fusarium* species.

Microscopic Morphology (Figs 8.41A to C)

- Numerous ascomata (perithecia) formed within 10-14 days that gave the colony a punctate appearance (incubated at light and dark conditions at 25°C).
- Microscopic studies revealed hyaline, elongated to cylindrical conidia aggregated in slimy heads on conidiogenous cells developing on undifferentiated hyphae.
- Conidia sizes varied from 5-10 μm in length 2-3 μm wide, and were mostly single celled or with one septum.
- Some conidia appeared slightly curved. Intercalary Chlamydospores were also observed.
- The microscopic morphology was consistent with *Acremonium* species.
- Perithecia were orange-brown in colour, subspherical (300-400 μm in diameter), multilayered and smoothed walled, each with an apical pore.
- Cylindrical asci, 90-110-10-12 μm in diameter, were present inside the ascomata, each containing 8 ascospores in a row. The ascospores were brownish, spherical to ellipsoidal, 10-15-8-12 μm, with thick roughened walls and no germ pore present.

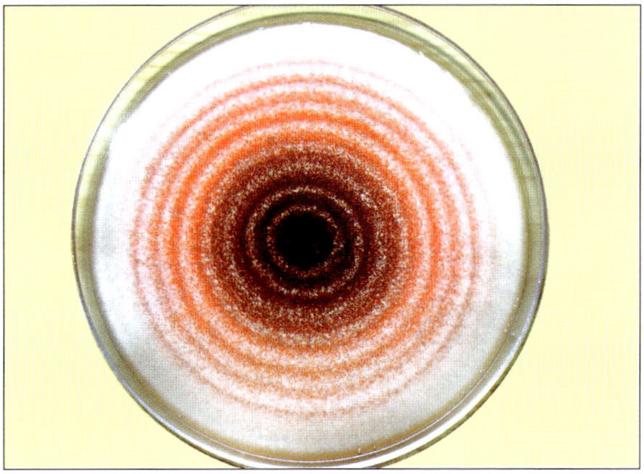

Fig. 8.40: Culture of *Neocosmospora vasinfecta* grown on potato agar at 25°C for 14 days

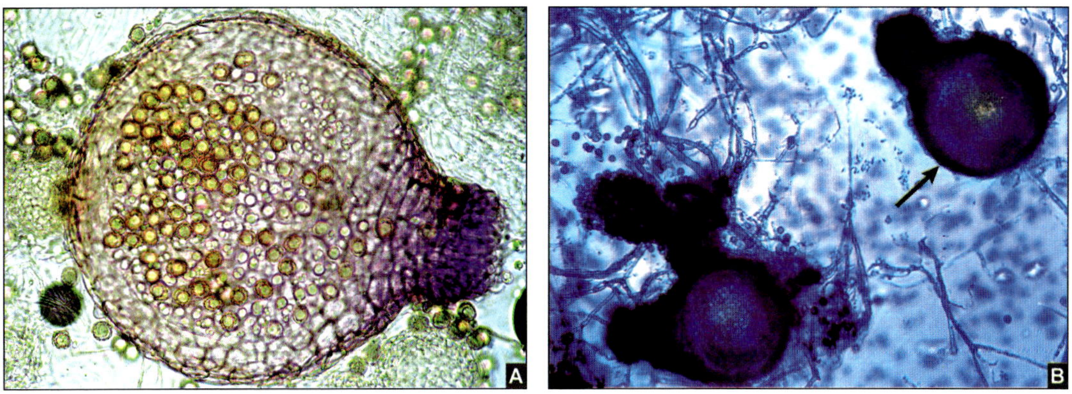

Figs 8.41A and B: Microscopically the perithecia are orange-brown in colour, subspherical (300-450 μm in diameter), smooth-walled and each has an apical pore

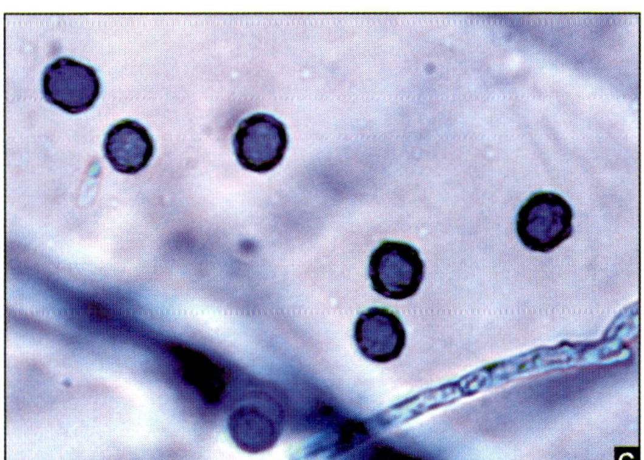

Fig. 8.41C: Ascospores are brownish, spherical to ellipsoidal and roughed cell walls (*Courtesy:* Manikandan P, et al. Corneal ulcer due to *Neocosmospora vasinfecta* in an immunocompetent patient. Med Mycol 2007;45:Sep 18; 1-6)

PAECILOMYCES

Pathogenicity

Paecilomyces species are rare pathogen reported into cause keratitis and endophthalmitis. They are usually present as a contaminant. Occasionally it has been reported as a pathogen in pulmonary infections, endocarditis, and sinusitis. Infections of cutaneous lesions have occasionally occurred after traumatic inoculation of the host, and *Paecilomyces* species have been associated with infections in patients who have had organ transplants.

Ecology

Cosmopolitan, isolated from soil and decaying plant material. Often implicated in decay of food products and cosmetics. Certain species parasitize insects.

Macroscopic Morphology (Fig. 8.42)

- Rapid growth
- Texture wooly to powdery
- Color rusty, olive brown, lilac, pinkish, beige or white on the surface, reverse pale.

Microscopic Morphology (Figs 8.43A and B)

- Hyphae septate, hyaline
- Conidiophores often branched
- Phialides thin and elongate at the tips, grouped in brush-like clusters at the ends of the conidiophores
- Conidia oval to fusoid, in long chains
- Chlamydospores sometimes present.

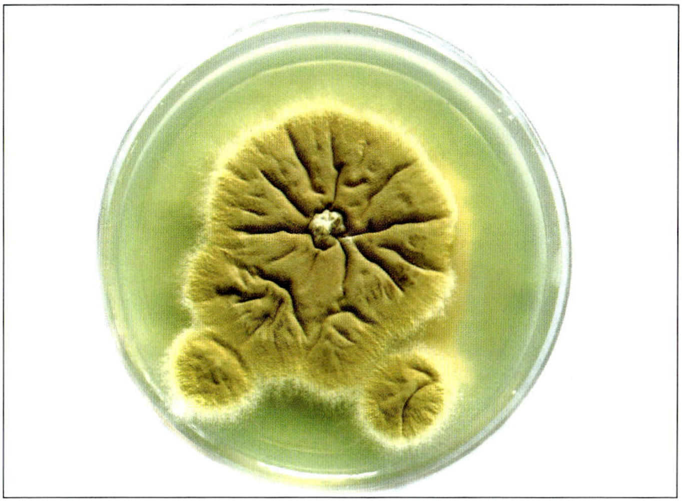

Fig. 8.42: *Paecilomyces* species growth on potato dextrose agar, 25°C, 5 days

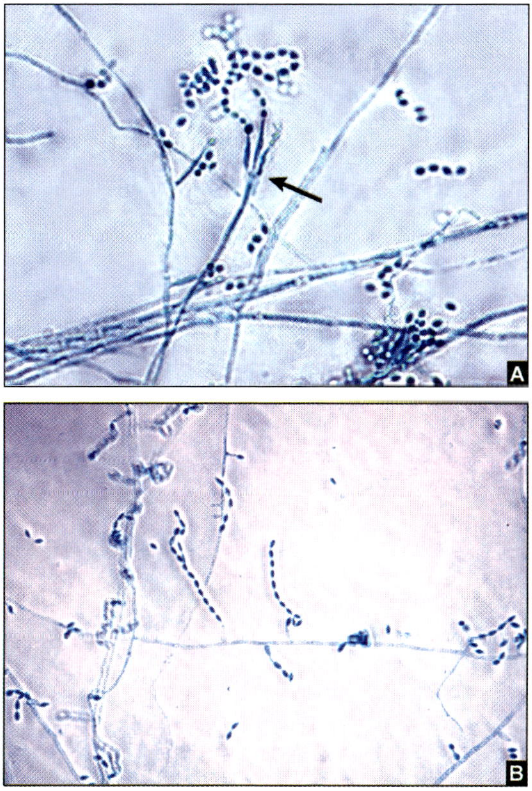

Figs 8.43A and B: Phialides with thinly tapered apices (→) and chains of oval conidia

PENICILLIUM SPP

Pathogenicity

Penicillium species are usually a contaminant or a secondary invader, but infections do occur. Seven of the approximately 900 species have been isolated as etiologic agents of infection. Pulmonary infections, keratomycosis, onychomycosis, external ear infections, cutaneous lesions, bladder infections and endocarditis due to *Penicililum* species have been reported with, in some cases, considerable doubt about the reliability of the report.

Ecology

Cosmopolitan, predominant in regions of temperature climate. Penicillia figure among the most common types of fungi isolated from the environment. Of the approximately 150 species recognized, some are frequently implicated in the deterioration of food products, where they may elaborate mycotoxins.

Macroscopic Morphology (Figs 8.44A and B)

- Growth moderately rapid to rapid
- Texture velvety to powdery
- Color green, blue grin, grey green, white, yellow or pinkish on the surface; reverse usually pale to yellowish, rough walled red or brown.

Microscopic Appearance (Fig. 8.45)

- For species other than *Penicillium marneffei*, septate hyaline hyphae (1.5 to 5 µm in diameter), simple or branched conidiophores, metulae, phialides, and conidia are observed. Metulae are secondary branches that form on conidiophores. The metulae carry the flask-shaped phialides.
- The organization of the phialides at the tips of the conidiophores is very typical. They form brush-like clusters which are also referred to as "penicilli". The conidia (2.5-5 µm in diameter) are round, unicellular, and visualized as unbranching chains at the tips of the phialides.
- In its filamentous phase, *Penicillium marneffei* is microscopically similar to the other *Penicillium* species. In its yeast phase, on the other hand, *Penicillium marneffei* is visualized as globose to elongated sausage-shaped cells (3 to 5 µm) that multiply by fission. *Penicillium marneffei* is easily induced to produce the arthroconidial yeast-like state by subculturing the organism to an enriched medium like BHI and incubating at 35°C, in which after a week, yeast-like structures dividing by fission and hyphae with arthroconidia are formed.

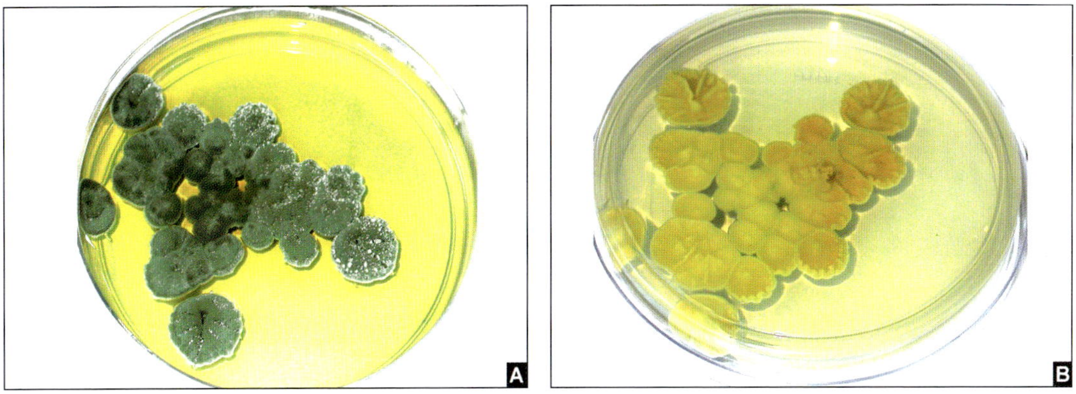

Figs 8.44A and B: *Penicillium* species growth on potato dextrose agar, 25°C, 7 days (**A**—Surface; **B**—Reverse)

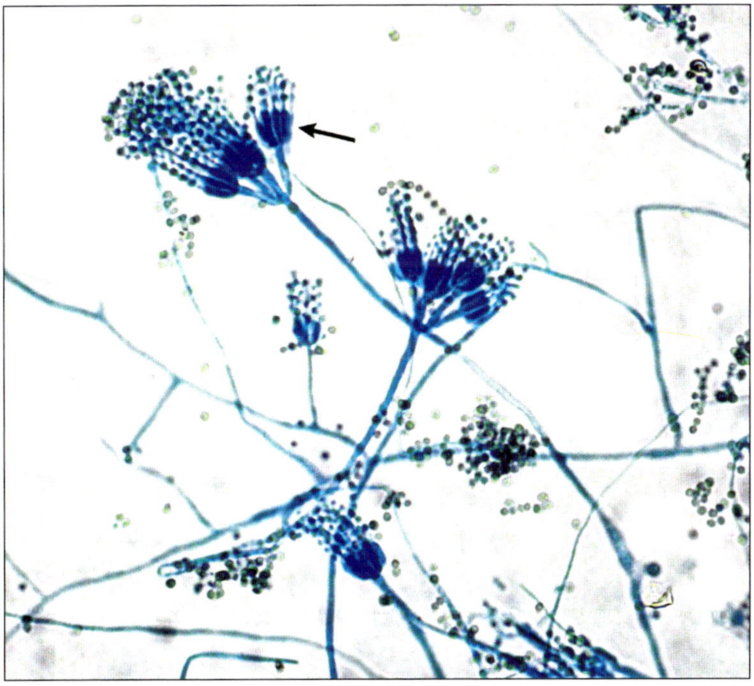

Fig. 8.45: *Penicillium* species. Phialides grouped in brush-like penicilli (→) and producing conidia in chains

PHIALOPHORA

Infections with *P.verrucosa* most often occur in people who work outdoors without protective clothing such as shoes and gloves. Repeated exposure and poor general health may contribute to development of the infection.

Pathogenicity

P. verrucosa can cause chromoblastomycosis or phaeohyphomycosis. The fungi are apparently introduced into host tissues through some minor injury where a contaminated splinter or thorn penetrates the skin. The infection spreads by autoinoculation and via the lymphatic system. *P. verrucosa* also includes several species causing diverse types of phaeohyphomycosis, presenting in the form of mycotic arthritis, subcutaneous cyst, osteomyelitis and cerebral or disseminated infection.

Ecology

Cosmopolitan, saprobes commonly isolated from decomposing wood, soil, and subaqatic debris in bodies of cold fresh water.

Macroscopic Morphology (Fig. 8.46)

- Colonies of *Phialophora* grow moderately slowly and attain a diameter of 2-3 cm following an incubation of 7 days at 25°C
- The texture is wooly to velvety and may be heaped and granular in some strains. From the front, the color is initially white and later becomes dark grey-green, brown or black. From the reverse, it is iron grey to black.

Microscopic Morphology (Fig. 8.47)

- Septate hyphae, phialides, and conidia are observed. The hyphae (up to 5 μm wide) are branched, and hyaline to brown. *Phialophora parasitica* typically produces hyphae with verrucose walls.
- In strains of *Phialophora*, conidial formation is *Phialophora* type. The phialides are usually flask- or bottle-shaped, pale brown to brown, and are terminally or laterally located on the hyphae. The length of the phialides may vary.
- The shape of the collarette varies from one *Phialophora* species to other. It is vase-shaped in *Phialophora verrucosa*, saucer- or vase-shaped in *Phialophora richardsiae*, and narrow with almost parallel contours in *Phialophora repens* and *Phialophora parasitica*.
- Conidia are unicellular, hyaline or brown, smooth, and round, oval or cylindrical in shape. These conidia accumulate in masses at the apices of the phialides with collarettes, giving the appearence of a vase of flowers.

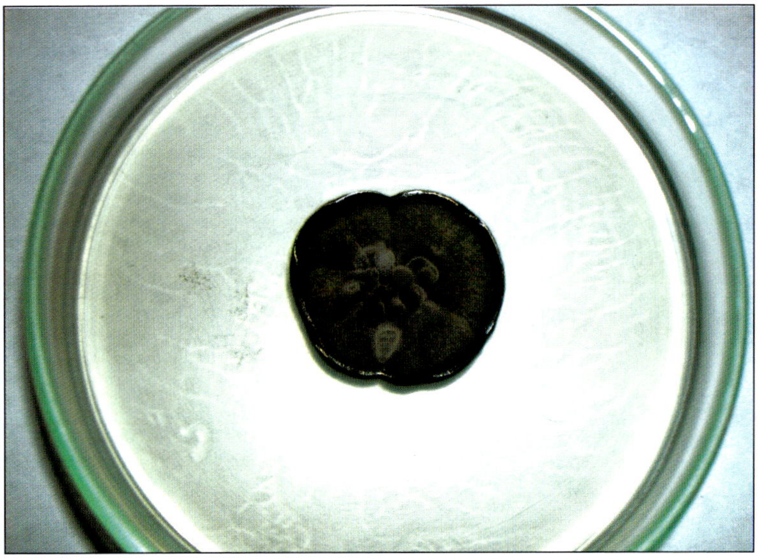

Fig. 8.46: *Phialophora verrucosa* growth on potato dextrose agar, 25°C, 7 days

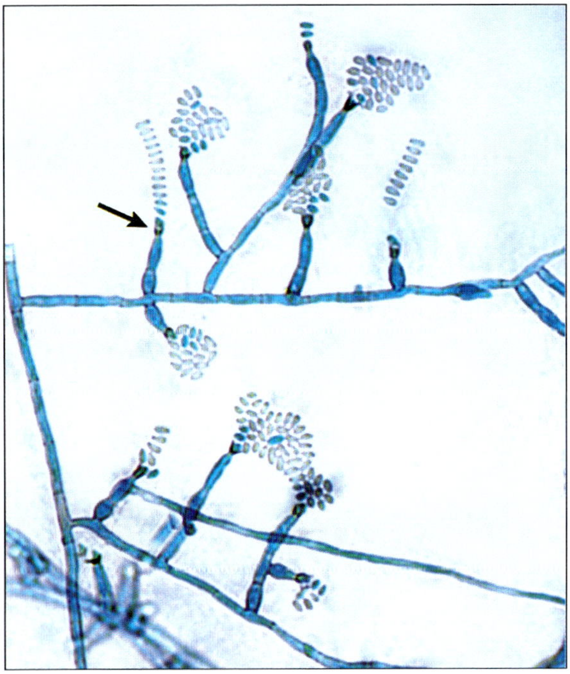

Fig. 8.47: Phialides with vase shaped (→) collarette

RHIZOPUS

Pathogenicity

Rhizopus is the principal agent of zygomycosis. This rapidly progressing infection is characterized by the necrosis of tissues and the production of infarcts in the brain, the lungs, and the intestines. Primarily, it is patients suffering from diabetic ketacidosis, malnutrition, severe burns, or immunocompromising conditions who are most at risk to develop this type of infection.

Ecology

Cosmopolitan, frequently isolated from soil and agricultural products (cereals, vegetables, etc). Certain species are plant pathogens.

Macroscopic Morphology (Fig. 8.48)

- Colonies of *Rhizopus* grow very rapidly, fill the Petri dish, and mature in 4 days.
- The texture is typically cotton-candy like. From the front, the color of the colony is white initially and turns grey to yellowish brown in time.
- The reverse is white to pale. Pathogenic species of *Rhizopus* can grow well at 37°C.

Microscopic Appearance (Figs 8.49A and B)

- Nonseptate or sparsely septate broad hyphae (6-15 µm in diameter), sporangiophores, rhizoids (root-like hyphae), sporangia, and sporangiospores are visualized.
- Sporangiophores are brown in color and usually unbranched.
- They can be solitary or form clusters.
- Rhizoids are located at the point where the stolons and sporangiophores meet. Sporangia (40-350 µm in diameter) are located at the tip of the sporangiophores. They are round with flattened bases.
- Apophysis is absent or rarely apparent and columellae are hemispherical. Sporangiospores (4-11 µm in diameter) are unicellular, round to ovoid in shape, hyaline to brown in color, and smooth or striated in texture.

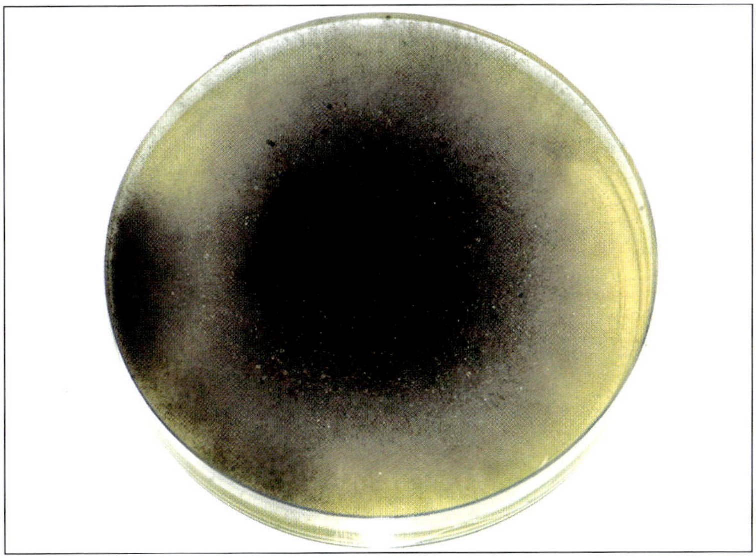

Fig. 8.48: *Rhizopus* growth on potato dextrose agar, 25°C, 5 days

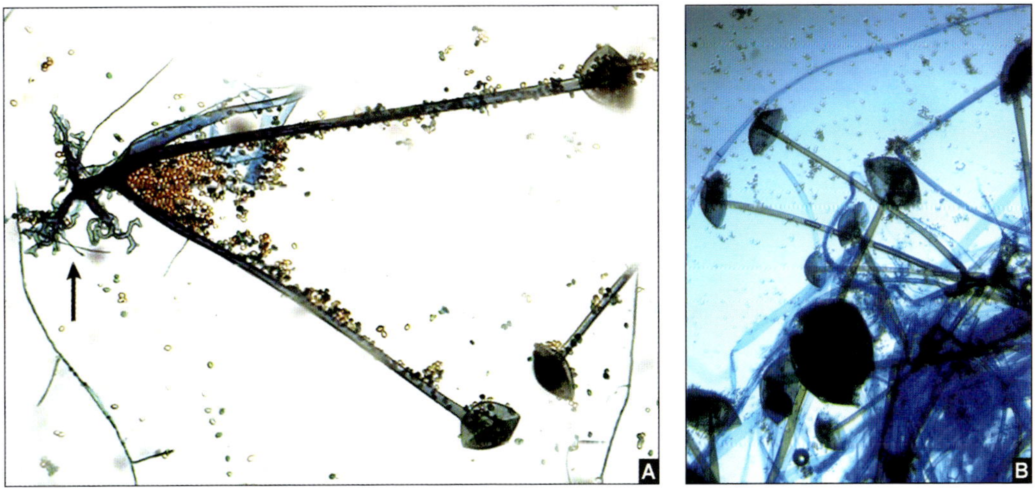

Figs 8.49A and B: *Rhizopus* spp. sporangiophores in tufts and rhizoids (→)

SCEDOSPORIUM APIOSPERMUM

Telemorph = *Pseudallescheria boydii*

Scedosporium apiospermum, previously known as *Monosporium apiospermum* is the anamorph of *Pseudallescheria boydii*, a fungus known for some time as *Petriellidium boydii* and *Allescheria boydii*.

Pathogenicity

Scedosporium apiospermum is a rare cause of endophthalmitis and keratitis. Ocular treatment of these pathologies usually proves ineffective due to the resistance of this fungus to the various antifungal agents currently marketed

An occasional agent of other infections including mycetoma, cutaneous or subcutaneous invasion, otitis, sinusitis, keratitis, endophthalmitis, pneumonia, endocarditis, meningitis, osteolyelitis, cerebral abscess and disseminated infection. Systemic infection is more commonly seen in the debilitated patient than in the normal host, but may occur in the latter under certain circumstances.

Ecology

It is a ubiquitous, earth-borne fungus commonly isolated from rural soils, from polluted water, from composts, and from manure of cattle and fowl.

Macroscopic Morphology

- Colonies of *Scedosporium apiospermum* grow rapidly at 25°C.
- The texture is wooly to cottony
- From the front, the color is initially white and later becomes dark gray or smoky brown. From the reverse, it is pale with brownish black zones (Figs 8.50A and B).

Microscopic Morphology (Fig. 8.51)

- Hyphae septate, hyaline
- Conidiophores with annellides simple or branced, little differentiated from vegetative hyphae

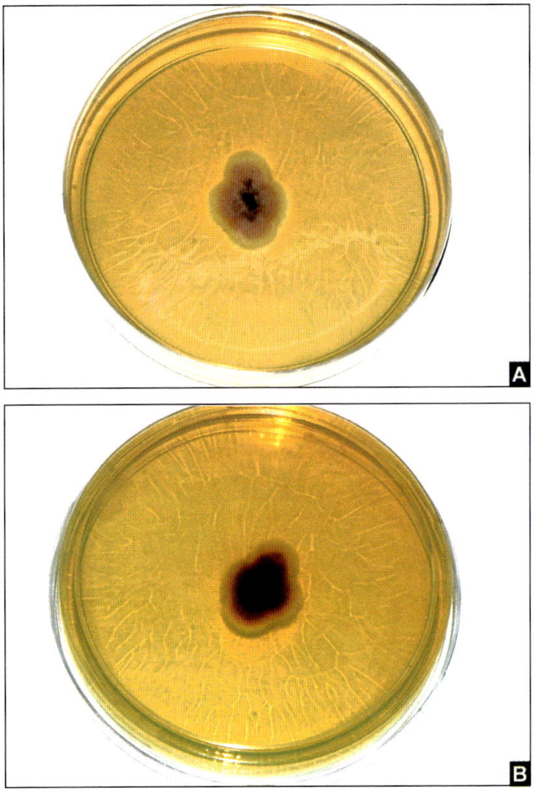

Figs 8.50A and B: *Scedopsorium apiospermum* growth on potato dextrose agar, 25°C, 5 days (**A**—Surface; **B**—Reverse)

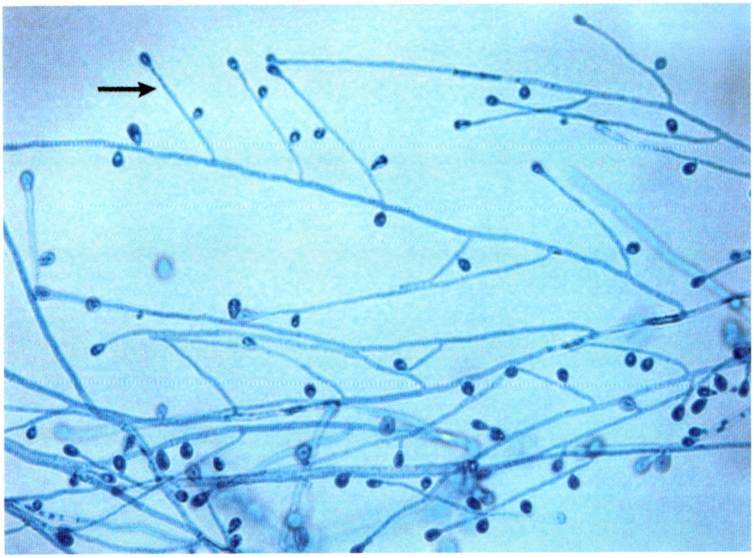

Fig. 8.51: *Scedosporium apiospermum* conidia at the tips of more or less elongate conidophores

- Conidia (annelloconidia) unicellular, pale brown, obovoid, with truncate bases, formed singly or in small clusters at the ends of conidiophores or from short annellidic necks arising directly from the hyphae [*Scedosporium* asexual state, always present (Figs 8.51 to 8.53)]
- Fascicles of conidiophores bound together in synnemata sometimes present (*Graphium* state)
- Brown cleistothecia often present after 2-3 weeks of incubation (sexual state *Pseudallescheria boydii*)
- Ascospores yellow-brown, ellipsoidal.

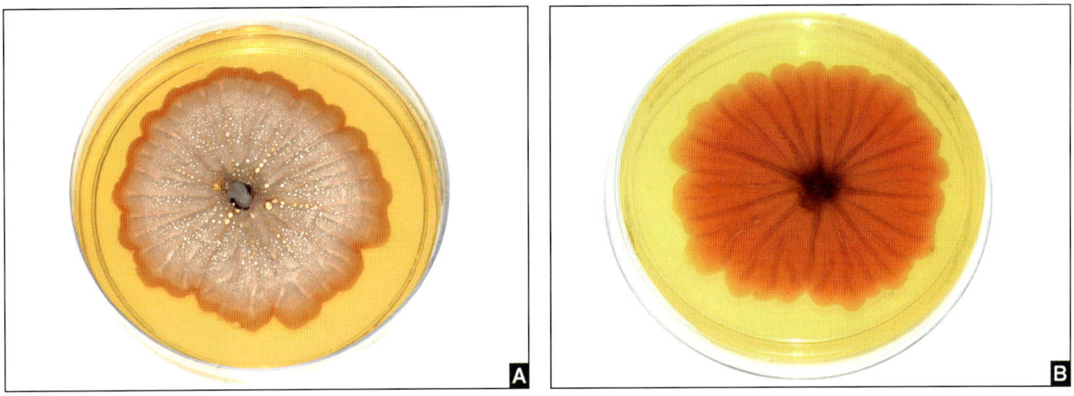

Figs 8.52A and B: *Scedopsorium prolificans* basally inflated annellides (Surface/Reverse)

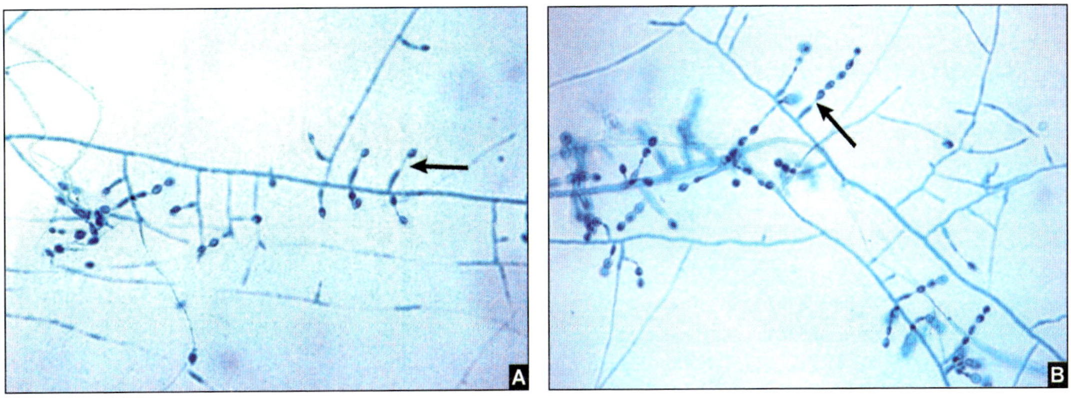

Figs 8.53A and B: *Scedosporium prolificans* - Basally inflated annllides (→)

CHAPTER

9

Molecular-based Diagnostics for Ocular Fungal Infections

POLYMERASE CHAIN REACTION (PCR)

PCR is rapid diagnostic technique to detect the infectious agents even in small volume of samples. PCR is typically used for one of the following scenarios:

1. The patient presents with signs and symptoms that are most likely an infection but a definitive diagnosis cannot be made.
2. When a patient does not respond appropriately to therapy, or
3. For confirmation of a diagnosis when a patient or
4. When the patient's natural history does not coincide with his or her clinical presentation.

Acquiring Sample for PCR Diagnostics

- Corneal scrapings
- Infected corneal button
- Aqueous and vitreous fluid, etc.

Typically, ophthalmic samples for PCR are collected in three ways. From least to most invasive, these include swab samplings of the external eye, an anterior chamber paracentesis, or a vitreous tap. The type of biopsy taken must be guided by disease suspicion, media opacity, structural parameters of the eye, coexistence of pathologic conditions, and the experience of the ophthalmologist in taking a biopsy from the vitreous or the anterior chamber.

Collection

All samples should be collected aseptically and placed into a sterile container. For a given PCR reaction volume, 5 to 10 μl of the patient sample is sufficient for amplification. Approximately 50 μl from an anterior chamber paracentesis is sufficient and should be immediately capped in a 1 ml sterile syringe. For vitrectomy samples, approximately 50-100 μl of a pre-infusion aspirate is collected in a sterile tube and capped upon collection. Vitrectomy samples are collected pre-infusion to prevent dilution of the pathogen DNA.

Placement of swab depends on disease suspicion. For suspicion of conjunctivitis, the swab is placed in the conjunctiva without touching the patient's external skin. For a corneal ulcer, the swab should be placed along the periphery of the ulcer, where the causative organism is most likely to be located. Once the sample is collected, the swab should be placed in a sterile tube containing 0.1 ml of a balanced salt solution. In the laboratory, the swab is "milked" and subsequently prepared for PCR.

Yield is not necessarily greatest with more invasive samples, such as aqueous or vitreous biopsies. For example, herpetic retinitis and CMV are better diagnosed with aqueous samples, whereas ocular toxoplasmosis and delayed-onset endophthalmitis is better diagnosed with a vitreous biopsy. External disease can be ideally diagnosed with swab samples.

Storage

Once obtained, both aqueous and vitreous specimens should be quick-frozen on dry ice or in liquid nitrogen and should remain so until the laboratory receives the sample. Freeze-thaw cycles are deleterious to the sample, degrading nucleic acids, particularly RNA. Swab samples should be stored at –70°C until the laboratory is ready to process them.

General Procedure

Polymerase chain reaction consists of three important steps:

1. Extraction of DNA from the standard strains of bacteria/fungi/viruses and clinical specimens
2. Amplification of the extracted DNA by PCR
3. Analysis of the amplified products by agarose gel electrophoresis.

DNA EXTRACTION PROTOCOLS—FROM CLINICAL SPECIMENS

Principle

Two methods for isolating DNA from different ocular samples are:

- Phenol chloroform extraction method
- Kit method (protocols followed as per the manufactures instructions, e.g. Qiagen, Germany).

PHENOL CHLOROFORM EXTRACTION METHOD

The cells containing DNA are chemically or physically lysed to release DNA, which is expected to have the nucleotide sequence or the region of interest.

1. Fluid samples includes extraction of DNA from aqueous humor, vitreous aspirate, cerebrospinal fluid and other body fluids. The fluid specimens are centrifuged at 3000 rpm for 15 minutes and deposit is used for DNA extraction in case of purulent specimens the required quantity is taken as such.
2. To 50 µl of the deposit of the fluid specimen equal volume of the lysis buffer solution (2 mg/ml of lysozyme in 20 mM Tris-Cl; ph- 8). 1 mM EDTA and 0.5% SDS) is added and incubated at 37°C for 1 hour.

3. Proteinase K is added to a final concentration of 200 µg/ml and incubated at 55°C to 60°C for 1 hour.
4. This is followed by addition of equal volume phenol: Chloroform: Isoamyl alcohol (25:24:1) and then sample is mixed gently 3-4 times and microfuged at 14,000 rpm for 15-20 mins. After that aqueous layer is separated into another sterile microfuge tube. If the aqueous layer is still turbid, another phnol:chloroform:isoamyl alcohol extraction is done.
   a. To the aqueous layer one tenth volume of 5 M Nacl and double the volume of 100% chilled ethanol is added and kept at –20°C for a minimum of 1 hour and a maximum of overnight.
5. To remove the salt from the precipitated DNA it is brought to room temperature, microfuged for 15 mins. The supernatant is discarded by just inverting the tube gently
6. Two hundred microlitres of 70% ethanol is added and is spun for 15 mins at 14,000 rpm. Supernatant is discarded and the pellet is again washed with 70% ethanol. The same step repeated thrice.
7. The tube is blotted on a blotting paper and mouth of the tube is covered with parafilm. Holes are made on the parafilm and tubes are kept at 37°C so that the ethanlol is completely removed by evaporation.
8. To the dried tube 30 µl of Milli Q water is added to dissolve the DNA and kept at –20°C

PCR CONDITIONS FOR OCULAR FUNGAL GENOME

PCR Primers

Primers specific for the Internal Transcribed Spacer Region (ITS) common to all medically important fungi as described by Lindsley et al is used.

Forward Primer ITS 1 : 5' TCC GTA GGT GAA CCT GCG G 3′

Reverse Primer ITS 4 : 5' TCC TCC GCT TAT TGA TAT GC 3′

The expected product is 601 bp in length. Primers can de custom synthesized by commercial companies.

PCR ASSAY

All the PCR reaction are carried out in a 50 µl reaction volume with 0.2 ml thin wall polypropylene tubes (Axygen Inc, CA, USA) using Biorad thermocycler (model PTC 200). The reagents added to the tube are 5 µl of 10X PCR buffer (15 mM $MgCl_2$, 500 mM KCl, 100 mM Tris-Cl and 0.01% gelatin), 8 µl of DNTP (1.25 mM of each DNTP) 10 pM of each nucleic acid primer, 1 U Taq Polymerase.

10 µl of DNA template and sterile water to make up the volume to 50 µl. PCR Amplification conditions are an initial step at 95°C for 5 minutes followed by 35 cycles carried out at 95°C for 30 minutes.

Step No.	*Description*	*Temperature*	*Time*
1	Initial denaturation	95°C	5 mins
2	Denaturation	95°C	30 seconds
3	Annealing	58°C	30 seconds
4	Extension	72°C	1 minute
5	Final extension	72°C	10 minutes

All PCR reactions include appropriate controls to exclude the possibility of DNA contamination. Visualization of the PCR product is done by subjecting 10 µl volume of the amplified reaction mixture to electrophoresis in Tris-borate buffer on 1.5% agarose gel incorporating 0.5 µg/ml ethidium bromide. The gel is examined on a UV transilluminator (302 nm) and photographed. The criterion for positivity is the presence of a 601bp band after amplification (Fig. 9.1).

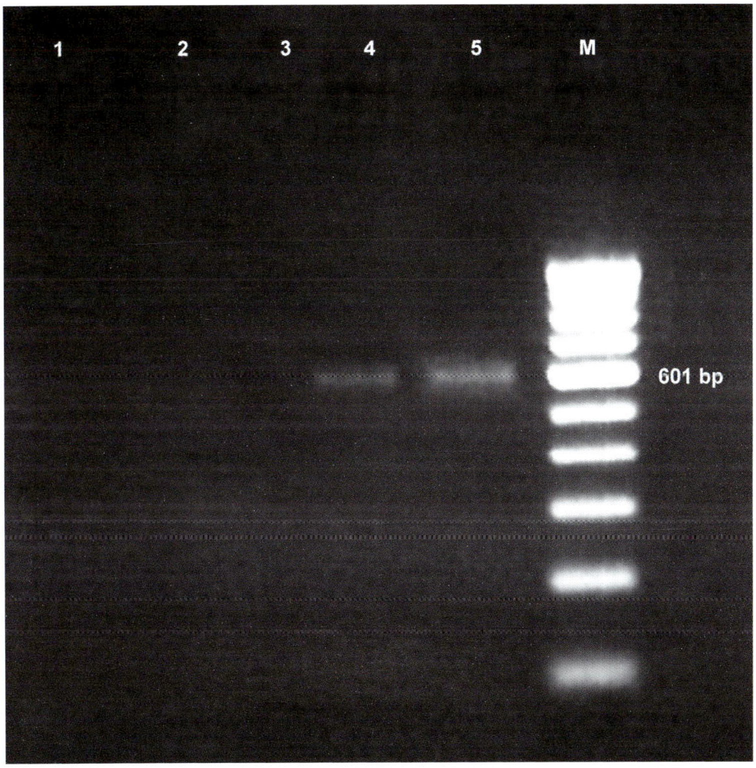

Fig. 9.1: 10 µl aliquots of amplified product with 2 µl loading buffer are run on a 1.5% agarose gel with ethidium bromide

Lane 1 shows PCR reagents
Lane 2 shows negative control
Lane 3 shows samplc
Lane 4 shows sample spiked with positive *Candida* DNA
Lane 5 positive control of *Candida* DNA showed specific band in 601bp product.

CHAPTER

10

Treatment of Fungal Keratitis

MEDICAL THERAPY

The antifungal agents available today are mostly fungistatic, requiring a prolonged course of therapy. Although models of *Aspergillus* and *Candida* have been established, there are no reliable animal models of *Fusarium* keratitis. Fungi considered to be ocular pathogens are rarely encountered among the systemic mycoses. Thus, the therapeutic principles valid for systemic fungal infections may not apply to the cornea (O'Day DM 1987). In vitro antifungal sensitivities often are performed to assess resistance patterns of the fungal isolate. However, in vitro susceptibility testing may not correspond with in vivo clinical response because of host factors, corneal penetration of the antifungal, and difficulty in standardization of antifungal sensitivities.

Polyenes

The polyenes include natamycin and amphotericin B. Polyenes disrupt the cell by binding to fungal cell wall ergosterol forming a polyenesterol complex that alters membrane permeability, depleting essential cellular constituents and are effective against both filamentous and yeast forms

Natamycin

Natamycin, available as 5% suspension (Natacyn, Alcon, Texas, USA; Natamet Sun Pharmaceuticals, Mumbai, India; Nata-Cipla Limited, Mumbai, India) is considered the drug of choice for filamentous fungi (O'Day DM 1987). Predominantly fungicidal tetraene polyene antibiotic, derived from *Streptomyces natalensis* Because of poor penetration, it is effective only in less severe superficial keratitis. (Prajna et al. 2003) conducted a prospective study comparing the efficacy of natamycin 5% and econazole 2% in 112 cases of culture-proved fungal keratitis and found no statistically significant difference between the two drugs. Moreover, natamycin is expensive; the supply is erratic, and often times difficult to obtain.

Amphotericin B

It is produced by a strain of *Streptomyces nodosus*; can be fungistatic or fungicidal and is available as a systemic preparation. To prepare the topical form, the compound is diluted with dextrose or distilled water to arrive at a 0.15 to 0.5% concentration (Fungizone, Sarabai Piramol, Vadodara,India).It can also be used through the subconjunctival (10 µg), intracameral (5-7.5 µg), intravitreal (10 µg) and intravenous routes (0.1 mg/kg body weight). The penetration of topically applied amphotericin B is poor in cornea with intact epithelium. Topical applications may cause punctate epithelial erosions. The spectrum of activity of amphotericin B covers Candida species (drug of choice) and *Aspergillus* sp. (Figs 10.1 and 10.2). It is not effective against *Fusarium* species (O'Day DM, et al 1986).

AZOLE COMPOUNDS

The azole compounds include triazoles: Econazole, clotrimazole, and the imidazoles: fluconazole, itraconazole and voriconazole. Azoles inhibit ergosterol synthesis at low concentrations, and at higher concentrations, they appear to cause direct damage to cell walls.

Triazole

Econazole

Econazole 1% in arachis oil is available as an ophthalmic preparation in India (Aurozole, Aurolab, Madurai, India). Prajna et al have found that the effect of this drug is equal to that of natamycin against filamentous fungi (Prajna et al 2003).

Clotrimazole

Clotrimazole is also available as a 1% topical preparation eye drops and in ointment form (Auroclot, Aurolab, Madurai, India) (Nistin-C, Jawa Pharmaceuticals, India). Mselle treated 12 patients with proven fungal keratitis with clotrimazole but suggested that clotrimazole as monotherapy is not an ideal choice (Mselle J 2001).

Imidazoles

Whereas the imidazoles; miconazole and ketoconazole, have less systemic toxicity, they are inferior to amphotericin B (Meunier-Carpentier F, 1983). Because of relatively reduced systemic toxicity and better corneal penetration, these compounds can be used systemically for keratomycosis. Thomas et al over a period of 10 years (1984-1994) treated 330 cultured-proved fungal keratitis cases with ketoconazole, itraconazole, amphotericin B, and natamycin and found that 69% of patients responded to ketoconazole, 66% to itraconazole, 53% to amphotericin B, and 56% to natamycin. In severe keratitis, it was less than 60% in all the groups. *Fusarium* is common in this region. Oral fluconazole and ketoconazole are absorbed systemically with good levels in the anterior chamber and the cornea; therefore, they should be considered in the management of deep fungal keratitis (Thomas PA, 2003).

Fluconazole

Fluconazole (Diflucon®, Pfizer NC, Zocon, Conflu), a fungistatic bitriazole is considered a topical and systemic agent in the treatment of fungal keratitis due to *Candida* and *Aspergillus* (Avunduk AM et al., 2003). However, fluconazole does not show encouraging results against *Aspergillus* species and *Fusarium* species (Rao SK et al., 1997). Panda et al from India compared the effect of natamycin 5%, polyhexamethylene biquanide (PHMB) 0.02%, 1% povidone iodine, and placebo in experimental *Aspergillus* keratitis in a rabbit model and concluded that PHMB was moderately effective and povidone iodine was not effective (Panda A et al, 2003).

Voriconazole

A new azole antifungal agent, voriconazole, is derived from fluconazole and shows a broader spectrum of activity against *Candida, Aspergillus, Scedosporium, Fusarium* and *Paecilomyces*. Jeu et al. described the mechanism of action. (Jeu L et al., 2003). As with other triazole antifungal agents, voriconazole exerts its effect primarily through inhibition of cytochrome P450-dependent 14_ sterol demethylase, an enzyme responsible for the conversion of lanosterol to 14_ demethyl lanosterol in the ergosterol biosynthetic pathway. In head-to-head comparative trials, voriconazole appeared to be as efficacious as amphotericin B for the treatment of invasive aspergillosis. In clinical studies, it was as efficacious as fluconazole and useful against fluconazole-resistant and itraconazole-resistant strains of *Candida*. Dose adjustment is recommended in patients with hepatic dysfunction. Eighty percent of this drug is hepatically eliminated. Shah et al. conducted an *in vitro* study to determine the activity of voriconazole compared with other polyene and imidazole antifungal agents against corneal isolates of *Scedosporium apiospermum* and found that the minimal inhibitory concentration of voriconazole was 0.5 µg/ml, a concentration lower than that of the other imidazoles (Shah KB et al, 2003).

Echinocandins

The echinocandins are caspofungin, micafungin, anidulafungin (Glucan synthesis inhibitors) Under new antifungal drugs, echinocandins are used for systemic mycoses.The target of the echinocandins is the synthetic cell wall enzyme complex -1,3- beta -D-glucan synthase. Caspofungin (Cansidas; Merck research labs) is a polypeptide antifungal related to pneumocandin B0 The antifungal spectrum is restricted to *Candida* species and *Aspergillus* species and is not active against *Fusarium* species (Denning DW, 2003).

SURGICAL THERAPY

Frequent corneal debridement with a spatula is helpful as it helps to reduce the bulk of the fungal organisms and enhance penetration of the topical antifungal agent. The use of *N-butyl* cyanoacrylate tissue adhesive in the management of corneal thinning or perforation associated with active fungal keratitis has been reported (Garg P et al, 2003). In a study of 73 patients, 63% showed resolution of infiltration with scar formation. Xie et al, have tried lamellar keratoplasty. Approximately one third of fungal infection fails to respond to medical

Amphotericin – B (5 μg/0.1ml)	
Volume & concentration	**Method**
50 mg vial 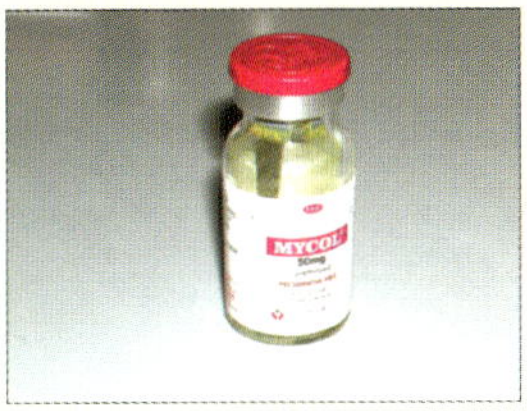	Available as 50 mg poser in a vial
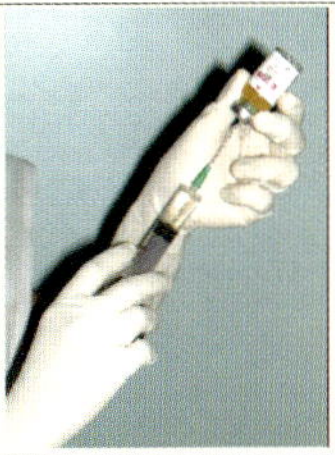	Reconstitute 10 ml of 5% dextrose (5 mg/ 5 ml) 50 mg in 10 ml or 5 mg in 1 ml 0.5 mg in 0.1 ml (0.5%)
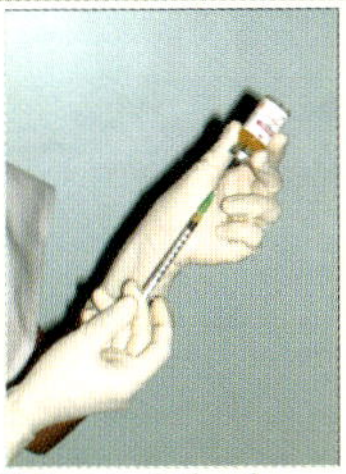 0.5 mg=0.1 ml (0.5%) 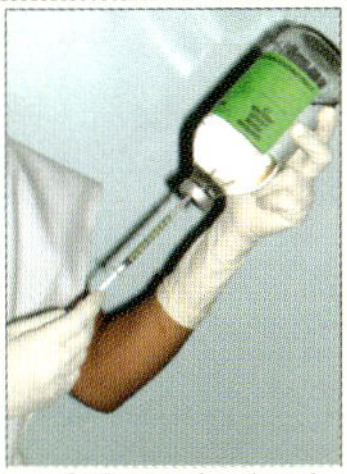 0.5 mg in 1 ml (0.05%)	Take 0.1 ml from 10 ml of Amphotericin B vial and make it to 1 ml 0.5 mg in 1 ml (0.05%) or 0.05 mg in 0.1 ml
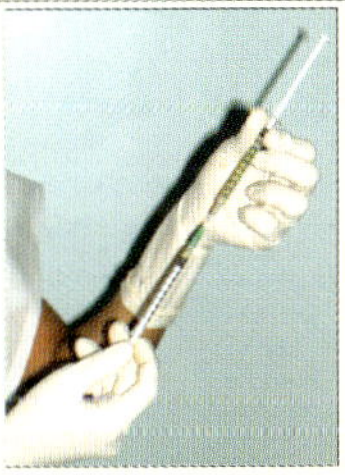 0.05 mg in 0.1 ml 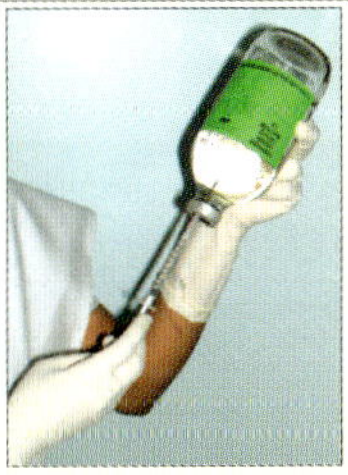 0.05 mg in 1 ml (0.005%)	Take 0.1 ml and remake it to 1 ml 0.05 mg in 1 ml (0.005%) or 0.005 mg in 0.1 ml 5 μg in 0.1 ml
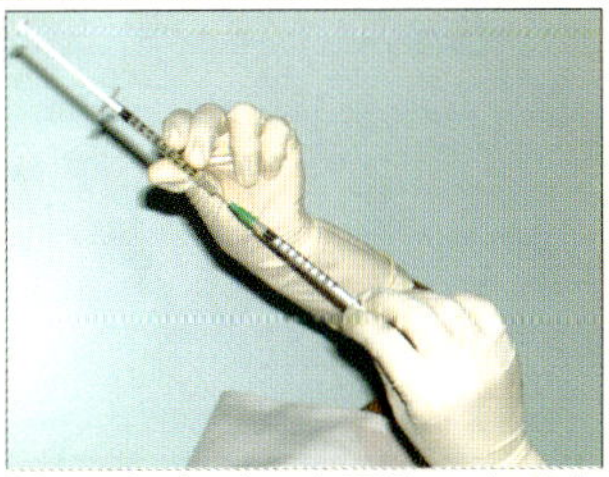 0.05 mg in 1 ml or 0.005 mg in 0.1 ml (5 μg in 0.1 ml)	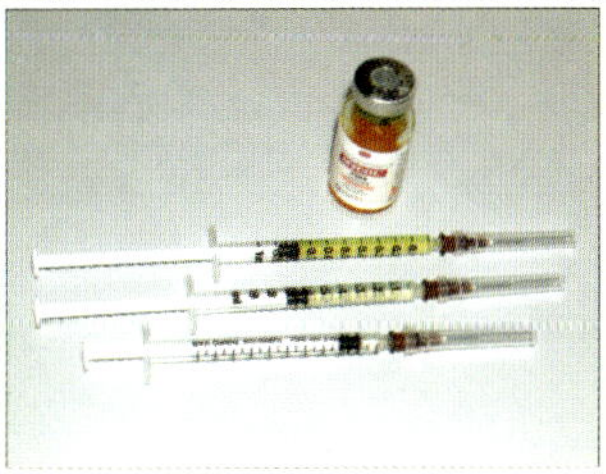 Take 0.1 ml of this for intravitreal injection 5 μg in 0.1 ml

Fig. 10.1: Amphotericin B preparation for intravitreal injection

Note: Reconstituted 10 ml solution can be used for one week; also the 1 ml remade up solution placed in a vial and used within a week (The vial must kept at –4°C)

Volume and concentration	Method
50 mg vial 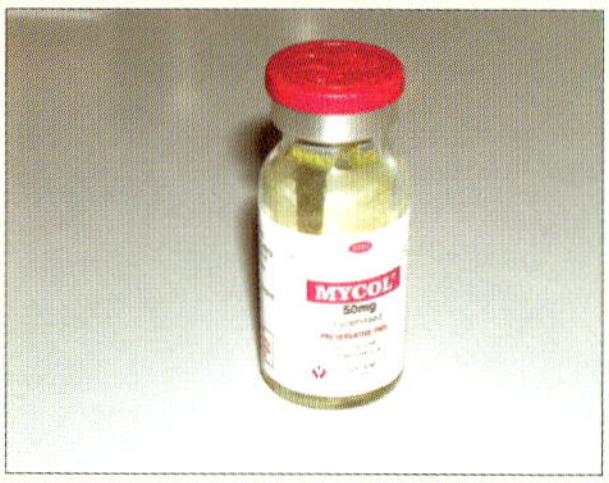	Available as 50 mg powder in a vial 50 mg/ vial

Once the Amphotericin B powder is reconstituted in water it will not be stable for a long time.

So it is better to prepare the minimal volume and keep it stored at —4°c. This should use with

50 mg powder can be divided and placed in 5 bottles in an sterile condition (10 mg each)

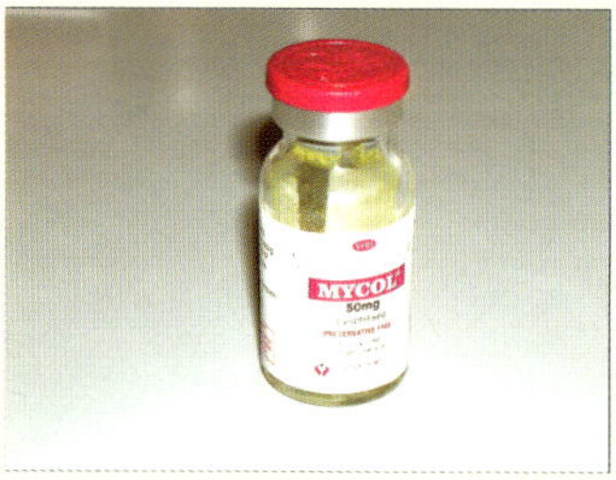

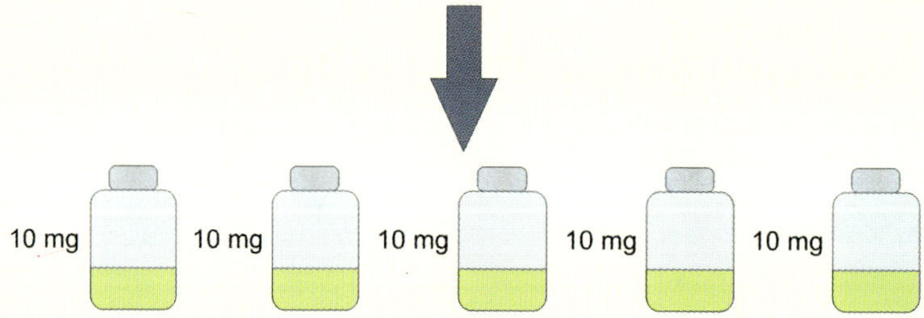

10 mg Amphotericin B powder each

Add 10 ml of sterile water 0.1% 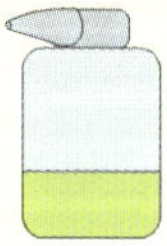 It must be stored in a dark bottle at —4°c. Use with in 2 or 3 days	Reconstitute 10 mg of powder in 10 ml of sterile water (10 mg / 10 ml) or 100 mg in 100ml 0.1 gm in 100 ml (0.1%)

Fig. 10.2: Amphotericin B preparation for topical application (0.1%)

treatment and may result in corneal perforation. (Xie et al, 2002). In these cases, a therapeutic penetrating keratoplasty is necessary. A small number of patients have been treated successfully with a conjunctival flap. The main goals of surgery are to control the infection and to maintain the integrity of the globe. Topical antifungal therapy, in addition to systemic fluconazole or ketoconazole, should be continued following penetrating keratoplasty. The use of topical corticosteroids in the postoperative period remains controversial.Structural integrity and eradication of sepsis is achieved in 80 to 90% of eyes and graft clarity in 36 to 89% (Panda A et al, 1991, Xie L et al, 2001 and Yao YF et al, 2003).

CONCLUSION

Current treatment methods frequently fail to preserve or restore vision after fungal keratitis. Although emerging antifungal agents show promise, therapeutic gaps will probably persist, and further development is necessary. Priorities should be given to develop and undertake drug trials against filamentous fungal keratitis.

Appendix

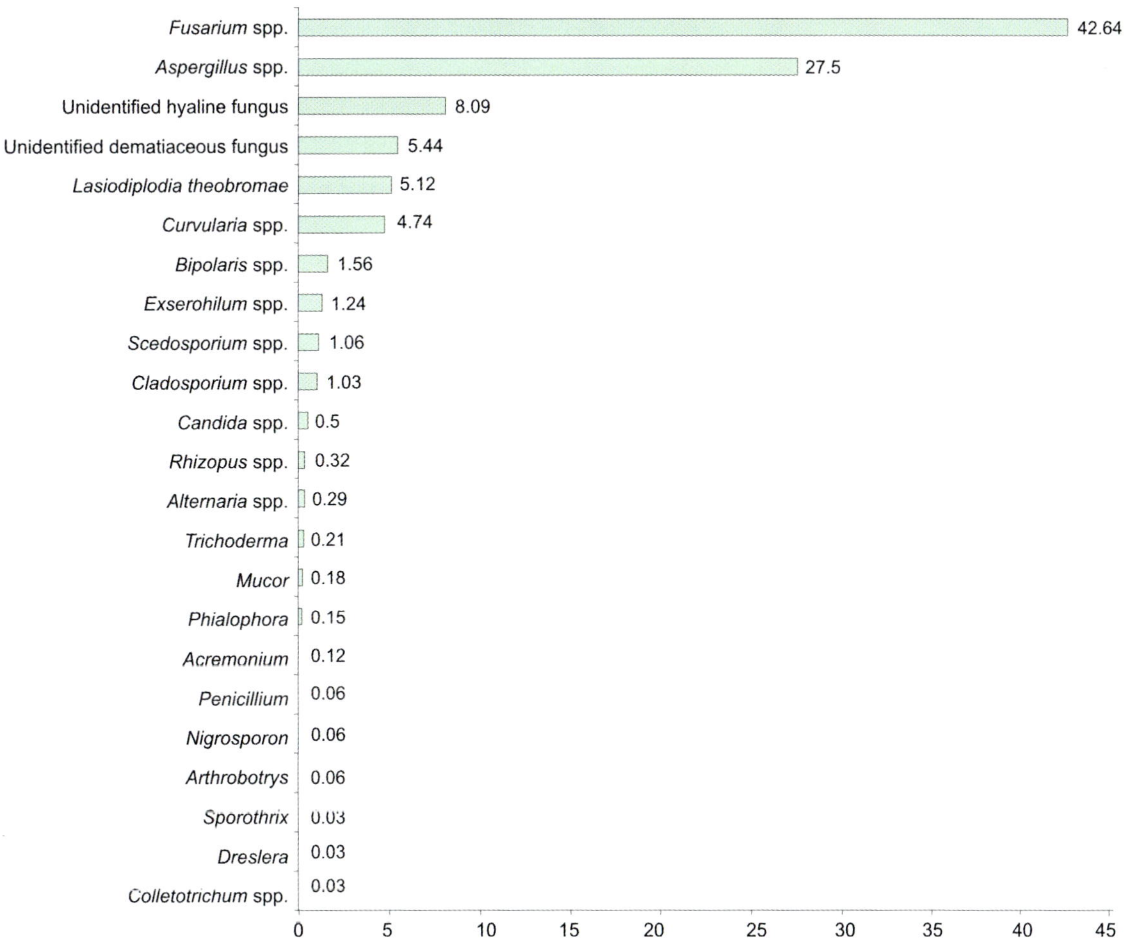

Diagram 1: Most common fungal pathogens isolated from corneal ulcers at the Department of Ocular Microbiology, Aravind Eye Hospital, Madurai (1997-2006)

Table 1: Prevalence of mycotic keratitis in India

No	Region	Author	Year	Total no. patients	No. positive for fungus	%	Major pathogens 1	Major pathogens 2
North Zone								
1	Chandigarh	Chander J, Sharma A	1994	730	61	8.4	*Aspergillus* 40.1%	*Fusarium* sps. 16.4%
2	Chandigarh	Talwar et al,	1978	100	34	34	*Aspergillus flavus* 17%	
3	Chandigarh	Chander J	1993	632	47	7.4	*Aspergillus fumigatus* 16%	
4	Patiala	Sharma et al	1981	100	19	19	*Aspergillus* spp. (52.6%)	
5	Delhi	Chowdhary A & Singh K	2005	485	191	39.4	*Aspergillus* 40.8%	*Curvularia* spp. 28.7%
6	Delhi	Saha R & Das S	2006	346	77	22.3	*Aspergillus* spp. 55.8%	*Candida* spp. 20.8%)
7	Kashmir	Bashkir G et al	2005	80	10	12.5	*Aspergillus fumigatus*	*Fusarium* sps.
West Zone								
8	Patna	Kumari N et a,	2002	204	76	37.3	*Aspergillus* spp. (52.3%)	*Candida* spp. (9.2%)
9	Udaipur	Kulshrestha et al.,	1973	52	23	44.2	*Aspergillus* spp. (35%)	
10	Mumbai	Deshpande et al,	1999	1010	367	36.3	*Aspergillus* spp. (59.7%)	*Candida* spp. (9.8%)
11	Aurangabad	Pichare A et al.,	2004	60	12	20	*Fusarium* spp. 6.6%	
East Zone								
12	Gauhati	Dutta et al.,	1981	100	32	32	*Aspergillus* spp. (69%)	
13	Goa	Verenkar MP et al,	1998	54	21	38.9	*Aspergillus* spp. (61.2%)	*Fusarium* spp. *Mucor* spp, *Penicillium* spp. 12.5%
14	Gangetic West Bengal	Basak SK et al.,	2005	1198	509	42.5	*Aspergillus* spp. 59.8%	*Fusarium* spp. 21.2%
South Zone								
15	Karnataka	Kotigadde et al,	1992	295	67	22.7	*Aspergillus fumigatus* (34.3%)	*Candida* spp. (19.4%)
16	Hyderabad (AP)	Reddy et al,	1972	600	36	6	*Aspergillus* sps. (6%)	

Contd...

Contd...

No	Region	Author	Year	Total no. patients	No. positive for fungus	%	Major pathogens 1	2
17	Hyderabad (AP)	Gopinathan U et al,	2002	3399*	1352	39.8	*Fusarium* spp. 37.2%	*Aspergillus* (30.7)
18	Hyderabad (AP)	Garg P et al,	2000	NM	557	NM	*Fusarium* spp. 37.6%	*Aspergillus* spp. 30.4%
19	Pondicherry	Dasgupta et al,	1973	175	50	28.6	*Aspergillus* spp. 50%	
20	Madurai	Srinivasan et al,	1997	434	139	32	*Fusarium* spp. 47.1%	*Aspergillus* spp. (16.1%)
21	Tirunelveli	Bharathi MJ et al,	2003	3183	1095	34.4	*Fusarium* spp. 42.8%	*Aspergillus* spp. 26%
22	Trichy	Leck AK et al,	2002	800	309	38.6	*Fusarium* spp. 39.9%	*Aspergillus* spp. 21.5%
23	Madras	Venugopal PL et al,	1989	698	322	46.1	*Aspergillus* spp. 43.8%	*Acremonium* spp
24	Madras	Sundaram et al,	1989	150	67	45	*Aspergillus* spp. 53%	*Fusarium* spp. and *Penicillium* spp. 12%
25	Pondicherry	Unpublished data	2006	781	317	40.6	*Fusarium* spp. 32%	*Aspergillus* (27.1%)

* Total number of culture proven cases
NM - Not mentioned

Table 2: Mycotic keratitis: a review of the world literature

No	Region	Author	Year	Total no. patients	% Fungi	Most common fungal isolates 1	2
Europe							
1	London	Coster et al	1981	67	3%	2 cases only	
2	London UK	Personal comm.	2001	72	3%	*Candida* sps. 58%	*Aspergillus flavus* 26%
3	Sweden	Neumann	1993	48	0%		
4	Brazil	Hofling-lima L	2005	14,391	296 (2.05%)	*Fusarium* (58.8%)	*Aspergillus* (12%)
5	Turkey	Yilmaz S	2007	620	22.3%	—	—
North America							
6	Florida	Liseagang	1980	663	20%	*Fusarium* 62%	*Candida* spp. 7.5%
7	Florida	Rosa	1994	125	Nm	*Fusaium* spp. 62%	*Candida* spp 12.5%
8	Philadelphia	Tanure	2000	24	Nm	*Candida albicans* 46%	*Fusarium* spp 25%
9	California	Ormerod	1987	227	11%	*Candida albicans* 4%	*Penicillium* spp 2%
10	Atlanta	Harris	1988	108	32	*Candida* spp (94%)	
11	New York	Ritterband DC		5083	1.2%	*Candida albicans* (48%)	
12	Northern USA Southern USA	O'Day	1987	33 285	Nm	*Candida* spp (42%) *Fusarium* spp (55 %)	*Aspergillus* sp. (30%) *Candida* spp (9.5%)
13	South America: Paraguay	Mino de Kaspar	1991	26	58%	*Fusarium* spp 42%	*Aspergillus* spp (19)
14	Paraguay	Laspina F	2004	660	26%	*Acremonium* spp 40%	*Fusarium* spp 15%
The Middle East							
15	Saudi Arabia	Khairallah	1992	191	14%	*Aspergillus* spp (41%)	*Fusarium* spp and *Candida albicans*
16	Iran	Tahereh Shokohi	2006	22	31.8%	*Aspergillus* spp (69%)	
	Tehran	Javadi	1996	23	83%	*Fusarium* 43%	*Aspergillus* 34.8%
	Rasht	Behboodi	1998	53	21%	*Cladosporium* 27%	*Candida albicans* 31.1%
	Tehran	Mirshahi	1999	35	83 %	*Fusarium* 34.5%	*Mucor* 31.1%
	Sari	Shokohi	1999	8	37.5 %	*Aspergillus* 33.3%	*Alternaria* 33.3%
	Mashhad	Berenji	2001	191	14 %	*Aspergillus* 55%	*Fusarium* 7%

Contd...

Contd...

No	Region	Author	Year	Total no. patients	% Fungi	Most common fungal isolates 1	2
Africa							
17	Ghana (Accra)	Hagan	1995	199	34%	*Fusarium* spp. 52%	*Aspergillus* spp. 15%
18	South Africa	Carmichael	1985	274	2%	*Curvularia* spp. 33%	
19	South Africa	Ormerod	1987	120	2.5%	*3 different isolates*	
20	Nigeria	Gugani	1976	59	Nm	*Fusarium* spp 36%	*Penicillium* spp. 29%
21	Tanzania	Mselle	1999	212	15%	*Fusarium* spp 75%	*Aspergillus* spp. 19%
22	Tanzania	TRG Poole	2002	24	50%	*Fusarium* spp. 20.5%	*Aspergillus* spp *Cladosporium* spp.
Australia & New Zealand							
23	Melbourne	Bhartiya P	2007	56	42.8%	*Candida albicans* (37.2%)	*Aspergillus fumigatus* (17.1%)
24	New Zealand	Wong T	2003	103	9%	*Yeast* 5%	*Filamentous fungi* 4%
South Asia							
25	North China	Xie L	2006	654	61.9%	*Fusarium* (73.3%)	*Aspergillus* spp. (12.1)
27	Thailand	Imwidthaya	1995	145	25%	*Aspergillus* spp. 34%	*Fusarium* spp 26%
28	Sri Lanka	Gonawardena	1994	66	33%	*Aspergillus* spp. 18%	*Single isolates*
29	Singapore	Wong	1997	29	NM	*Fusarium* spp. 52%	*A flavus*17%
30	Hong Kong	Houang	2001	223	2%	*Fusarium* spp. 60%	
31	Japan	Toshida H	2007	122	6.1%	*Candida* spp.	
32	Taiwan	Fong CF	2004	453	13.5%	*Fusarium* spp. 4% *Candida* spp. 4%	*Aspergillus* spp. 2%
33	Nepal, Dharan	Khana	2001	86	44%	*Aspergillus* spp. 60%	*Fusarium* spp. 13%
34	Nepal, Kathmandu	Upadhyay	1991	405	17%	*Aspergillus* spp. 47%	*Candida* spp. 13%
35	Nepal	Chaudhary	1999	110	8%	*Rhizopus* spp. 22%	NM
36	Bangladesh	Rahman	1998	63	NM	*Aspergillus* spp. 35%	*Fusarium* spp. 35%
37	Bangladesh	Dunlop	1994	66	36%	*Aspergillus* spp. 40%	*Fusarium* spp. 21%
38	Bangladesh	Williams	1991	127	34%	*Aspergillus* spp. 49%	*Fusarium* spp. 28%
39	Bangladesh	Williams	1987	33	21%	*Aspergillus* spp. 29%	*Fusarium* spp. 14%

NM - Not mentioned

Bibliography

1. Agarwal V, Biswas J, Madhavan HN, Mangat G, Reddy MK, et al. Current perspectives in Infection. Indian J Ophthalmol 1994;42:171–91.
2. Alexandrakis G, Jalali S, Gloor P. Diagnosis of Fusarium keratitis in an animal model using the polymerase chain reaction. Br J Ophthalmol 1998;82:306–11.
3. Asbell P, Stenson S. Ulcerative keratitis. Survey of 30 years laboratory experience. Arch Ophthalmol 1982;100:77-80.
4. Avunduk AM, Beuerman RW, Warnel ED, et al. Comparison of efficacy of topical and oral fluconazole treatment in experimental Aspergillus keratitis. Curr Eye Res 2003;26:113–17.
5. Bharathi MJ, Ramakrishnan R, Samala Vasu, Meenakshi, et al. Epidemiological characteristics and laboratory diagnosis of fungal keratitis. A three year study. Indian J Ophthalmol 2003;51:315–21.
6. Bhartiya P, Daniell M, Constantinou M, Islam FM, Taylor HR. Fungal keratitis in Melbourne. Clin Experiment Ophthalmol 2007;35(2):124-30
7. Brod RD, Flynn HW, Clarkson JG, Pflugfelder SC, Culbertson WW, Miller D. Endogenous Candida endophthalmitis. Management without intravenous amphotericin B. Ophthalmology 1990;97(5):666-72; disc: 672-4.
8. Byrne KA, Burd EM, Tabbara KF, Hyndiuk RA. Diagnostic Microbiology and Cytology of the Eye. Butterworth–Heinemann. Newton, Chapter 5 & 6. MA. I edn. 1995.
9. Chander J, Sharma A. Prevalence of fungal corneal ulcers in northern India. Infection 1994;22:207–9.
10. Chang CW, Ho CK, Chen ZC, et al. Fungi genus and concentration in the air of onion fields and their opportunistic action related to mycotic keratitis. Arch Environ Health, 2002;57:349-54.
11. Chitra Rajalakshmi P, Lalitha P. Textbook of Ocular Microbiology–Aravind Eye Hospital & Postgraduate Institute of Ophthalmology, Madurai 2006.
12. Choi DM, Goldstein MH, Salierno A, et al. Fungal keratitis in a daily disposable soft contact lens wearer. Contact Lens Association of Ophthalmologists Journal 2001;27:111-12.
13. Coster DJ, Wihelmus J, Peacock J, et al. Suppurative keratitis in London. The cornea in health and diseases. VIth Congress of the European Society of Ophthalmology 1981;40:395-8.
14. Coster DJ, Wilhelmus K, Peacock J, et al. Suppurative keratitis in London. Fourth Congress of the European Society of Ophthalmology, Royal Society of Medicine, International Congress and Symposium Series No. 40. London 1981;395–98.
15. Denning DW. Echinocandin antifungal drugs. Lancet 2003;4:362:1142–51.
16. DK Mendiratta, D Thamke, A K Shukla, P Narang. Keratitis due to Colletotrichum dematium – A case report Indian Journal of Medical Microbiology 2005;23(1):56-58.
17. Dongx, Xie L, Shi W, et al. Penetrating keratoplasty in management of fungal keratitis. Chin J Ophthalmol 1994;35:386-87.
18. Dunlop AA, Wright ED, Howlader SA, et al. Suppurative corneal ulceration in Bangladesh: a study of 142 cases examining the microbiological diagnosis, clinical and epidemiological features of bacterial and fungal keratitis. Aust N Z J Ophthalmol 1994;22:105–10.
19. Dunlop AAS, Wright E, Newman M, et al. Causes of suppurative keratitis in Bangladesh. Aus NZ J Ophthalmol 1994;22:105–10.
20. Dursun D, Fernandez V, Miller D, et al. Advanced Fusarium keratitis progressing to endophthalmitis. Cornea 2003;22:300–03.
21. Dutta LC, Dutta D, Mohanty P, Sharma J. Study Of Fungal Keratitis. Indian J Ophthalmol 1981;29:407-40.
22. Florakis GJ, Moazami G, Schubert H, et al. Scanning slit confocal microscopy of fungal keratitis. Arch Ophthalmol 1997;115:1461–63.

23. Fong CF, Tseng CH, Hu FR, Wang IJ, Chen WL, Hou YC. Clinical characteristics of microbial keratitis in a university hospital in Taiwan. Am J Ophthalmol 2004;137(2):329-36.
24. Forster RK, Rebell G. The diagnosis and management of keratomycoses: I. Cause and diagnosis. Arch Ophthalmol 1975;93:975–78.
25. Garg P, Gopinathan U, Choudhary K, et al. Keratomycosis: clinical and microbiologic experience with Dematiaceous fungi. Ophthalmology 2000;107:574–80.
26. Garg P, Gopinathan U, Nutheti R, et al. Clinical experience with N-butyl cyanoacrylate tissue adhesive in fungal keratitis. Cornea 2003;22:405–08.
27. Garg P, Rao GN. Corneal ulcer – Diagnosis and Management. Community eye health 1999;12:21-24.
28. Gaudio PA, Gopinathan U, Sangwan V, et al. Polymerase chain reaction based detection of fungi in infected corneas. Br J Ophthalmol 2002;86:755–60.
29. Germain GS, Summerbell R. Identifying Filamentous fungi – A Clinical Laboratory Handbook. Star Publishing Company, California. I edn. 1996.
30. Gonawardena SA, Ranasinghe KP, Arseculeratne SN, et al. Survey of mycotic and bacterial keratitis in Sri Lanka. Mycopathologia 1994;127:77-81.
31. Gopinathan U, Garg P, Fernandes M, et al. The epidemiological features and laboratory results of fungal keratitis: a 10-year review at a referral eye care center in South India. Cornea 2002;21:555–59.
32. Hagan M, Wright E, Newman M, et al. Causes of suppurative keratitis in Ghana. Br J Ophthalmol 1995;79:1024-8.
33. Höfling-Lima AL, Forseto A, Duprat JP, Andrade A, Souza LB, Godoy P, Freitas D. [Laboratory study of the mycotic infectious eye diseases and factors associated with keratitis][Article in Portuguese] Arq Bras Oftalmol. 2005;68(1):21-7. Epub 2005 Mar 30.
34. Houang E, Lam D, Fan D, et al. Microbial keratitis in Hong Kong: relationship to climate, environment and contact lens disinfection. Trans R Soc Trop Med Hyg 2001;95:361–7.
35. Imwidthaya P. Mycotic keratitis in Thailand. J Med Vet Mycol 1995;33:81-2.
36. Jeu L, Piacenti FJ, Lyakhovetskiy AG, Fung HB. Voriconazole. Clin Ther 2003,25:1321–81.
37. Josep Cano, Josep Guarro, Josepa Gene. Molecular and morphological identification of Colletotrichum species of clinical interest. J Clin Microbiol 2004;42(6):2450-54.
38. Khairallah SH, Byrne KA, Koornhof HJ. Fungal keratitis in Saudi Arabia. Doc Ophthalmol 1992;79:269-76.
39. Khanal B, Kaini KR, Deb M, et al. Microbial keratitis in eastern Nepal. Tropical Doctor 2001;31:168–9.
40. Kredics L, Varga J, Kocsubé S, Dóczi I, Samson RA, Rajaraman R, Narendran V, Bhaskar M, Vágvölgyi C, Manikandan P. Case of Keratitis Caused by Aspergillus tamarii. J clin Microbiol. 2007;45(10):3464-7. Epub 2007 Aug 15.
41. Kredics L, Varga J, Kocsubé S, Dóczi I, Samson RA, Rajaraman R, Narendran V, Bhaskar M, Vágvölgyi C, Manikandan P. Case of Keratitis Caused by Aspergillus tamarii. J Clin Microbiol 2007;45(10):3464-7. Epub 2007 Aug 15.
42. Kunimoto DY, Sharma S, Garg P, et al. Corneal ulceration in the elderly in Hyderabad, SouthIndia. Br J Ophthalmol 2000;84:54-9.
43. Lalitha P, Prajna NV, Kabra A, Srinivasan M. Risk Factors for Treatment Outcome in Fungal Keratitis Ophthalmology 2006;113:526-53.
44. Leck AK, Thomas PA, Hagan M, Kaliamurthy J, Ackuaku E, et al. Aetiology of suppurative corneal ulcers in Ghana and South India, and epidemiology of fungal keratitis. Br J Ophthalmol 2002;86:1211-15.
45. Liesegang TJ, Forster RK. Spectrum of microbial keratitis in South Florida. Am J Ophtahlmol 1980;90: 38-47.
46. Mahajan VM. Ulcerative keratitis: an analysis of laboratory data in 674 cases. J Ocul Ther Surg 1985;4: 138-41.
47. Manikandan P, HF Vismer, L Kredics, I Dóczi, WFO Marasas, M Bhaskar, R Anita, R Revathi, V Narendran D. Corneal ulcer due to Neocosmospora vasinfecta in an immunocompetent patient. Med Mycol 2007;45: 1-6.

48. Manikandan P, Vismer HF, Kredics L, Dóczi I, Marasas WF, Bhaskar M, Anita R, Revathi R, Narendran V. Corneal ulcer due to Neocosmospora vasinfecta in an immunocompetent patient. Med Mycol 2007;Sep 18:1-6.
49. Mathews MS, Kuriakose T. Keratitis due to Cephaliophora irregularis Thaxter. Jnl of Med Vet Mycol 1995;33:359-60.
50. Meunier-Carpentier F. Treatment of mycoses in cancer patients. Am J Med 1983;24:74-79.
51. Mino de Kaspar H, Zoulek G, Paredes ME, et al. Mycotic Keratitis in Paraguay. Mycosus 1991;34:251-4.
52. Mselle J. 1991 Use of topical clotrimazole in human keratomycosis. Ophthalmologica 2001;215:357-60.
53. O'Brien TP. Bacterial keratitis, Chapter 94. In: Cornea: Cornea and External Diseases, clinical Diagnosis and management. Krachmer JH, Mannis MJ, Holland EJ, Eds. (St. Louis, Mosby): 1997;1139-89.
54. O'Day DM, Head WS, Robinson RD, et al. Corneal penetration of topical amphotericin B and natamycin. Curr Eye Res 1986;5:877-82.
55. O'Day DM. Selection of appropriate antifungal therapy. Cornea 1987;6:238-45.
56. Panda A, Ahuja R, Biswas NR, et al. Role of 0.02% polyhexamethylene biguanide and 1% povidone iodine in experimental Aspergillus keratitis. Cornea 2003;22:138-41.
57. Panda A, Sharma N, Das G, et al. Mycotic keratitis in children: epidemiologic and microbiologic evaluation. Cornea 1997;16:295-99.
58. Panda A, Vajpayee RB, Kumar TS. Critical evaluation of therapeutic keratoplastyin cases of keratomycosis. Ann Ophthalmol 1991;23:373-76.
59. Periman LM, Harrison DA, Kim J. Fungal keratitis after photorefractive keratectomy: delayed diagnosis and treatment in a co-managed setting. J Refract Surg 2003;19:364-66.
60. Prajna NV, John RK, Nirmalan PK, et al. A randomised clinical trial comparing 2% econazole and 5% natamycin for the treatment of fungal keratitis. Br J Ophthalmol 2003;87:1235-37.
61. Prajna NV, Rao Rema A, Mathen Minu M, Prajna L, George C, Srinivasan M. Simultaneous bilateral fungal keratitis caused by different fungi. Indian J Ophthalmol 2002;50:213-14.
62. Rao SK, Madhavan HN, Rao G, et al. Fluconazole in filamentous fungal keratitis. Cornea 1997;16:700.
63. Ritterband DC, Seedor JA, Shah MK, Koplin RS, McCormick SA. Fungal keratitis at the new york eye and ear infirmary. Cornea 2006;25(3):264-7.
64. Rodriguez-Ares T, De Rojas Silva V, Ferreiros MP, Becerra EP, Tome CC, Sanchez-Salorio M. Acremonium keratitis in a patient with herpetic neurotrophic corneal disease. Acta Ophthalmol Scand 2000;78(1):107-9.
65. Rosa RH, Miller D, Alfonso EC. The changing spectrum of fungal keratitis in South Florida. Ophthalmology 1994;101:1005-13.
66. Saha R, Das S. Bipolaris keratomycosis. Mycoses 2005;48(6):453-5.
67. Samir H. Khairallah, Kathleen A Byrne, Khalid F. Fungal keratitis in Saudi Arabia. Documenta Ophthalmologica 1992;79(3).
68. Shah KB, Wu TG, Wilhelmus KR, et al. Activity of voriconazole against corneal isolates of Scedosporium apiospermum. Cornea 2003;22:33-36.
69. Sharma S, Srinivasan M, George C. The current status of Fusarium species in mycotic keratitis in South India. J Med Microbiol 1993;11:140-47.
70. Smith EF. Wilt disease of cotton, watermelon and cowpea. USDA Bull 1899;17:1-53.
71. Srinivasan M, Gonzales CA, George C, Cevallos V, et al. Epidemiology and aetiological diagnosis of corneal ulceration in Madurai, South India.Br J Ophtahlmol 1997;81:965-71.
72. Srinivasan M. Fungal keratitis, Curr Opin Ophthalmol 2004;15:321-27.
73. Subbannaya Kotigadde, Ballai M, Jyothiralatha, et al. Mycotic keratitis: a study in coastal Karnataka. Indian J Ophthalmol 1992;40:31-3.
74. Sundaram BM, Badrinath S, Subramanian S. Studies on mycotic keratitis. Mycosus 1989;32:568-72.
75. Tanure MA, Cohen EJ, Sudesh S, et al. Spectrum of fungal keratitis at Wills Eye Hospital Philadelphia, Pennsylvania. Cornea 2000;19:307-12.
76. Tanure MA, Cohen EJ, Sudesh S, et al. Spectrum of fungal keratitis at Wills Eye Hospital, Philadelphia, Pennsylvania. Cornea 2000;19:307-12.

77. Thomas PA, Kuriakose T. Keratitis due to Arthrobotrys oligospora Fres. 1850. Jnl of Med Vet Mycol 28: 47-50.
78. Thomas PA. Current perspectives on ophthalmic mycoses. Clin Microbiol Rev 2003;16:730-97.
79. Thomas PA. Fungal infections of the cornea. Eye 2003;17:852-62.
80. Tuli SS, Yoo SH. Curvularia keratitis after laser in situ keratomileusis from a feline source. J Cataract Refract Surg 2003;29:1019-21.
81. Upadhyay MP, Karmacharya PC, Koirala S, et al. Epidemiologic characteristics,predisposing factors, and etiologic diagnosis of corneal ulceration in Nepal. Am J Ophthalmol 1991;15:92-99.
82. Varenkar MP, Shubhangi B, Pinto MJM, Naik PA. Study of mycotic keratitis in Goa. Indian J Med Microbiol 1998;16:58-60.
83. Venugopal PL, Venugopal TL, Gomathi A, et al. Mycotic keratitis in Madras. Indian J Pathol Microbiol 1989;32:190-7.
84. Verma S, Tuft SJ. Fusarium solani keratitis following LASIK for myopia. Br J Ophthalmol 2002;86:1190-91.
85. Vincent M. Borderie,Bourcier TM, Poirot JP, Marie Baudrimon, et al. Endophthalmitis after Lasiodiplodia theobromae corneal abscess Graefe's Archive for Clinical and Experimental Ophthalmology 1997;235:(4) 259-61.
86. Whitcher JP, Srinivasan M, Upadhyay MP. Corneal blindness: a global perspective. Bull World Health Organisation 2001;79:214-21.
87. Whitcher JP, Srinivasan M. Corneal ulceration in the developing world: a silent epidemic. Br J Ophthalmol 1997;81:622-23.
88. Wong T, Ormonde S, Gamble G, McGhee CN. Severe infective keratitis leading to hospital admission in New Zealand. Br J Ophthalmol. 2003;87(9):1103-8.
89. Wong TY, Fong KS, Tan DTH. Clinical and microbial spectrum of fungal keratitis in Singapore: a 5 – year reterospective study. Int Ophthalmol 1997;21:127-30.
90. Xie L, Dong X, Shi W. Treatment of fungal keratitis by penetrating keratoplasty. Br J Ophthalmol 2001;85:1070-74.
91. Xie L, Shi W, Liu Z, Li S. Lamellar keratoplasty for the treatment of fungal keratitis. Cornea 2002;21:33-37.
92. Xie L, Zhong W, Shi W, Sun S. Spectrum of fungal keratitis in north China. Ophthalmology 2006;113(11):1943-8. Epub 2006 Aug 28.
93. Yao YF, Zhang YM, Zhou P, et al. Therapeutic penetrating keratoplasty insevere fungal keratitis using cryopreserved donor corneas. Br J ophthalmol 2003;87:543-47.
94. Yilmaz S, Ozturk I, Maden A. Microbial keratitis in West Anatolia, Turkey: a retrospective review. Int Ophthalmol 2007;27(4):261-8. Epub 2007.

Useful websites for Medical Mycology:

- www.drfungus.org
- www.mycobank.org
- www.isham.org
- www.mycologyonline.org
- www.aspergillus.org.uk
- www.fungusfocus.com
- www.mycology.adelaide.edu.au
- www.clinical-mycology.com
- www.nlm.nih.gov/medlineplus/fungalinfections

Glossary

Canaliculitis	Inflammation of the tubular passage in the eye lid that connects the punctum to the lacrimal sac
Cellulitis, orbital	Inflammation of the orbital tissues resulting from infection that extends from the nasal sinuses or teeth, by metastatic spread of infection elsewhere, or from introduction of bacteria caused by orbital trauma
Cellulites, preseptal	Inflammation of the subcutaneous tissue of the eyelids, contained in the spaces defined by the fibrous attachments of the skin to the superior and inferior orbital rims and posteriorly by the orbital septum
Conjunctivitis	Inflammation of the delicate membrane tissue lining the eyelids and eyeball connected to the sclera and corneal tissue
Corneal ulcer	Local defect or excavation of the corneal tissue caused by invasion by microorganisms, trauma or hypoxia
Decryocystitis	Infection of the lacrimal sac, often secondary to nasolacrimal duct obstruction.
Endophthalmitis	Inflammation of the ocular cavities and intraocular tissues restricted to the uveal tract, vitreous body and retina.
Hypopyon	Accumulation of inflammatory cells and exudates in the interior chamber, producing a fluid level macroscopically visible in the inferior portion
Iritis	Inflammation of the iris
Keratitis	Inflammation of the cornea
Keratomycosis	Fungal infection of the cornea
Keratoplasty	Corneal grafting; transplantation of donor corneal material to replace scar tissue that interferes with vision
Trachoma	A chronic conjunctivitis caused by *Chlamydia trachomatis* and characterized by progressive exacerbations and remissions with follicular subconjunctival hyperplasia, corneal vascularization, and cicatrization of the conjunctiva, cornea and lids.
Uveitis	Inflammation of the uvea

A

Acropetal
Having the youngest conidia at the apex of a chain.

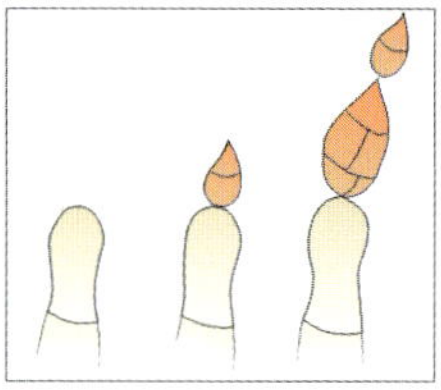

Acicular
Slender, gradually becoming narrower towards the apex.

Aculeate
Bearing narrow spines.

Aerial hyphae
Hyphae that grow above the agar surface.

Anamorph (anatomic morphology)
The asexual form of the fungus that is recognized solely based on its anatomic morphology.

Annelide
A conidiogenous cell that gives rise to successive conidia in a basipetal manner. The apex of an annellide becomes longer and narrower as each subsequent conidium is formed and released. An apical ring composed of outer cell wall material remains as each conidium is released.

Anneloconidia
A conidium formed by an annellide.

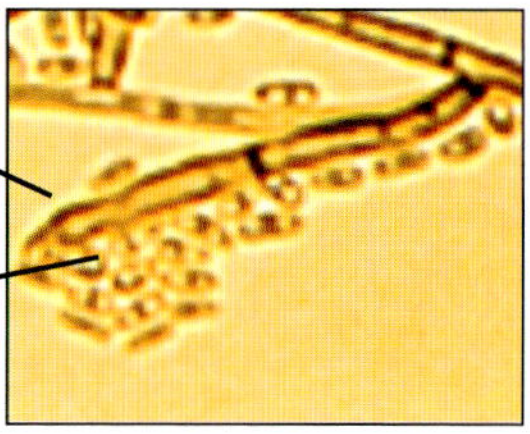

Annular frill
A ring or skirt like portion of cell wall material at the base of a conidium that remains when the conidium separates from its conidiophore.

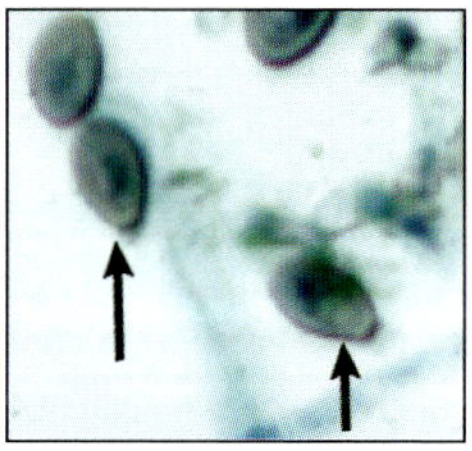

Apothecium
A disk-shaped or cup-shaped ascocarp of some ascomycetous fungi.

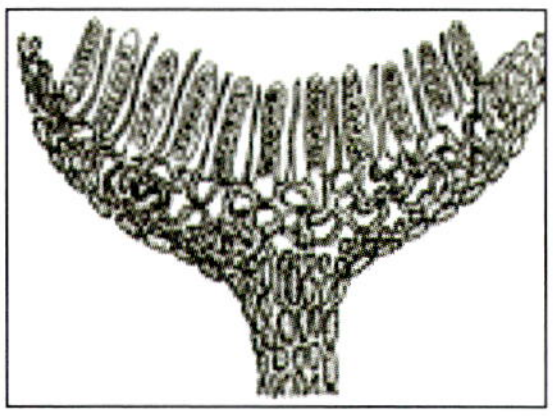

Arthroconidia (pl. arthroconidia)
A conidium formed by the modification of a hyphal cell(s) and then released by the fragmentation-lysis of a disjunctor cell or by fission through a thickened septum.

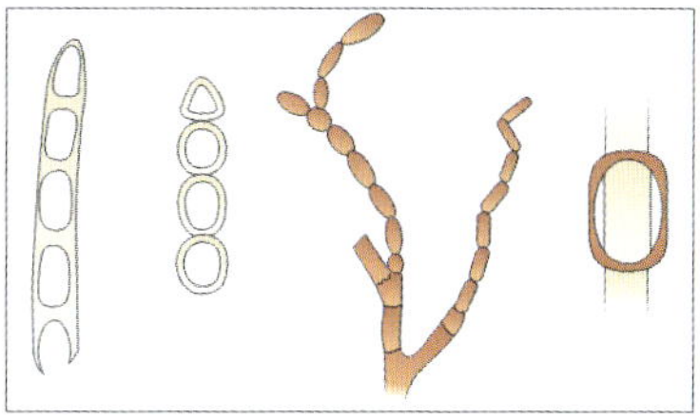

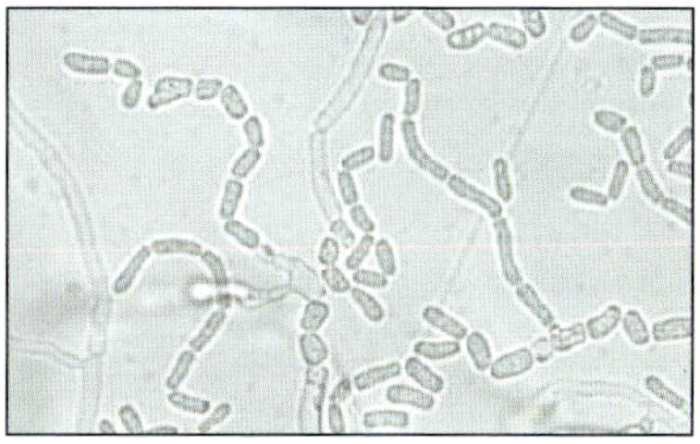

Ascospore
A haploid sexual spore that is formed by free-cell formation in an ascus following karyogamy and meiosis.

Ascus (pl. asci)
A sac like cell in which ascospores are produced after karyogamy and meiosis.

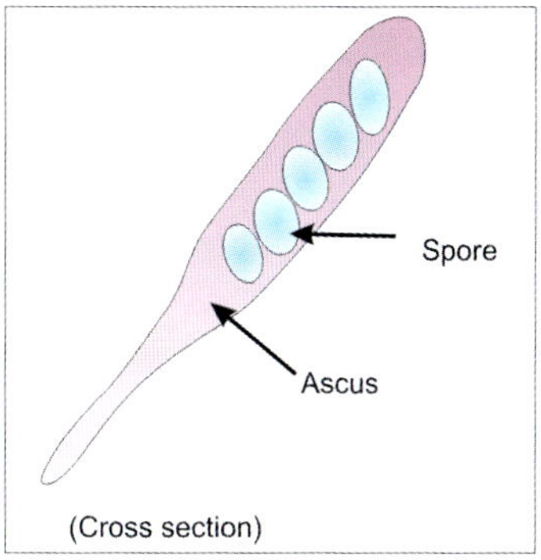

Assimilation
The utilization of nutrients for growth with oxygen serving as the final electron acceptor.

Awl shaped
Shaped like an awl; broad at the base tapering gently upward to a slender stiff point.

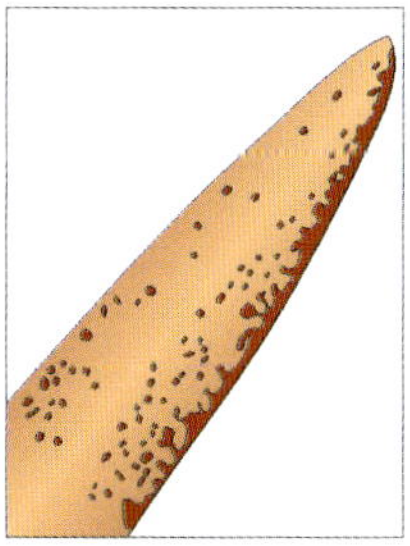

B

Ballistoconidium (pl. ballistoconidia)
Conidium formed on spine-like outgrowth of a cell, forcibly discharged by a droplet mechanism, e.g. sporobolomyces.

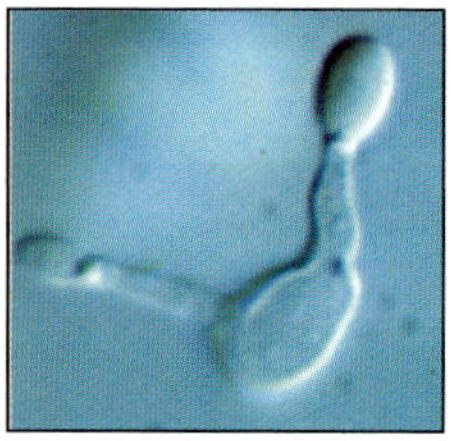

Balloon form
Pertaining to a large globose conidium formed by some dermatophytes.

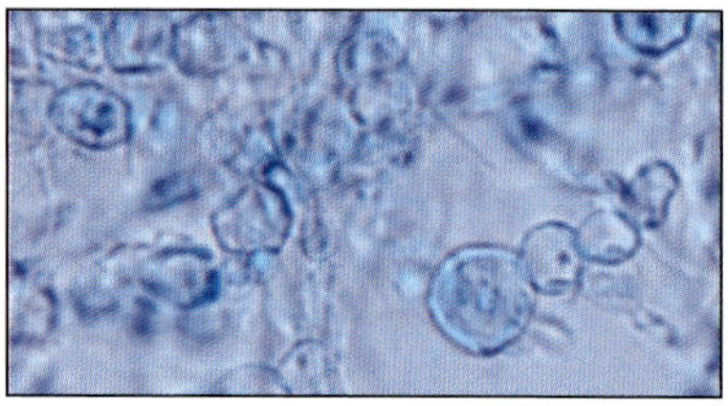

Basidiospore
A haploid sexual spore formed on a basidium following the process of karyogamy and meiosis.

Basidium (pl. basidia)
A specialized cell that gives rise to basidiospores. Basidia are characteristic of the Basidiomycetes.

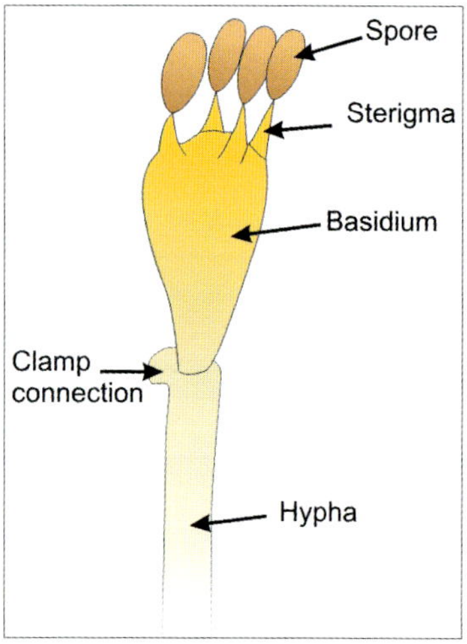

Basipetal
Having the youngest conidia at the base of a chain.

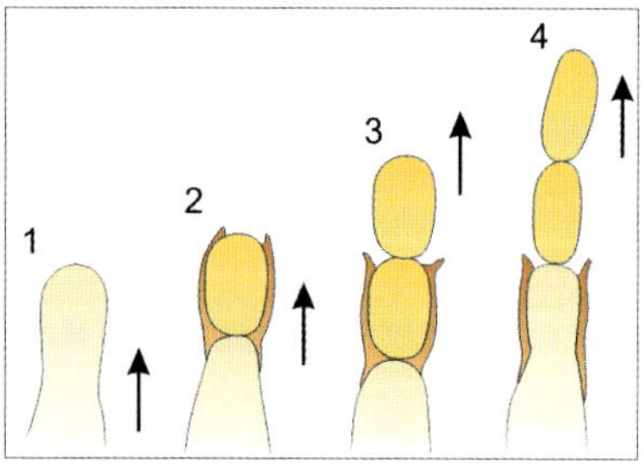

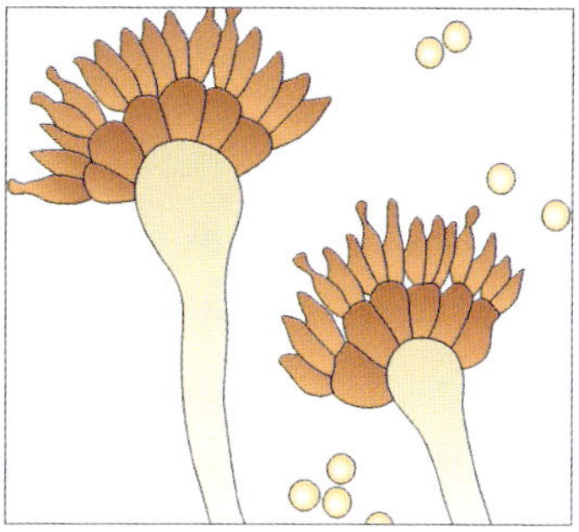

Bipolar budding
The development of conidia at both ends of the parent cell.

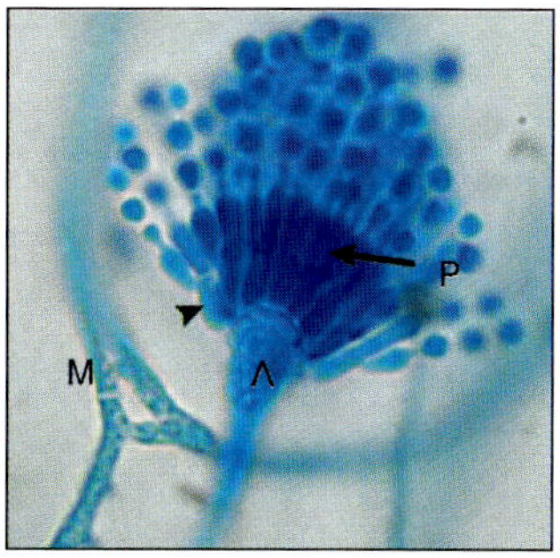

Biseriate
Having phialides(P) arising from metulae(M) on the vesicles of species of *Aspergillus*.

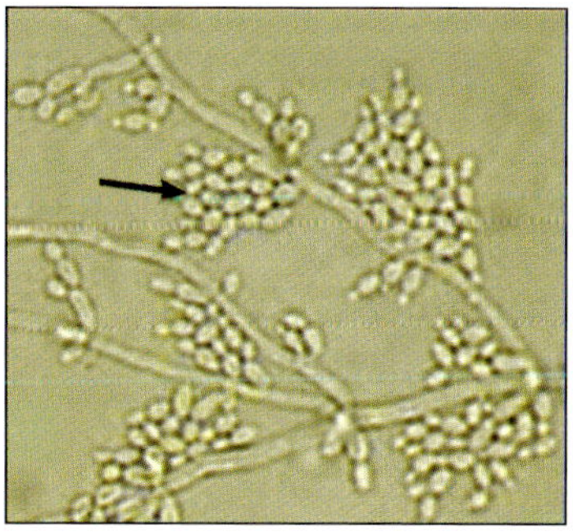

Blastoconidia/Blastospore
A conidium that is blown out from part of its parent cell and is typically released by fission through a thickened basal septum.

Budding
Asexual formation of small, rounded outgrowths from a parent cell.

C

Capsule
A hyaline mucopolysaccharide sheath around the cell wall of certain yeasts, e.g. *Cryptococcus* and *Rhodotorula*.

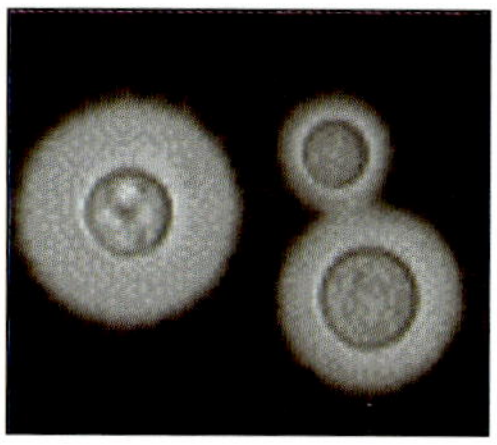

Carry over
Indigenous substances stored within the cells of inoculum, nutrients in the original culture medium, or both. These substances support growth of the test isolate in an assimilation study

Chlamydoconidium/Chlamydospore
A rounded, enlarged conidium that usually has a thickened cell wall and functions as a survival propagule.

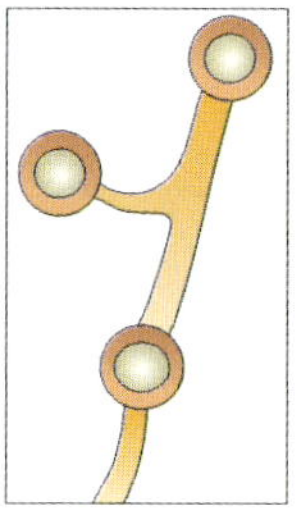

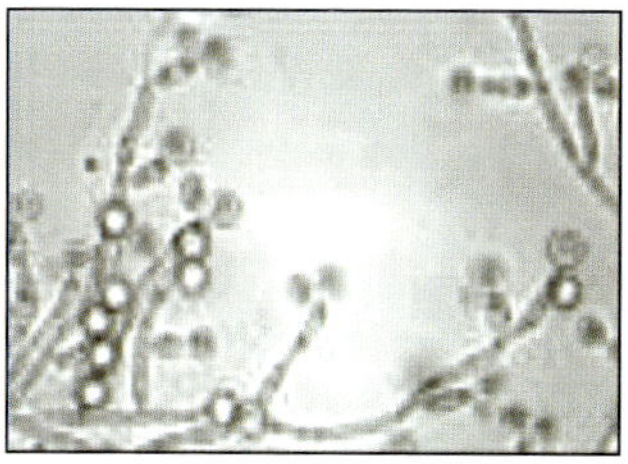

Circinate
Coiled into a complete or partial ring.

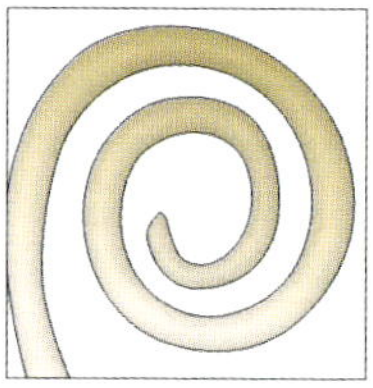

Clamp connection
Hyphal outgrowth in Basidiomycota which, at cell division, makes a connection between the two cells forming a by-pass around the septum to allow the migration of a nucleus.

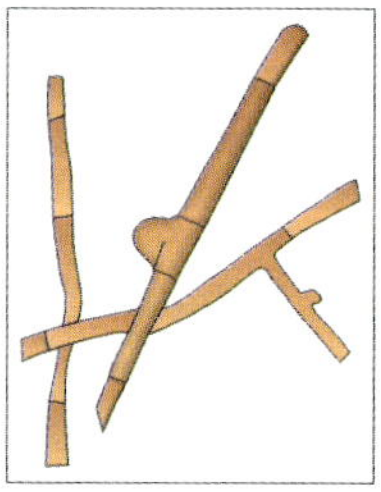

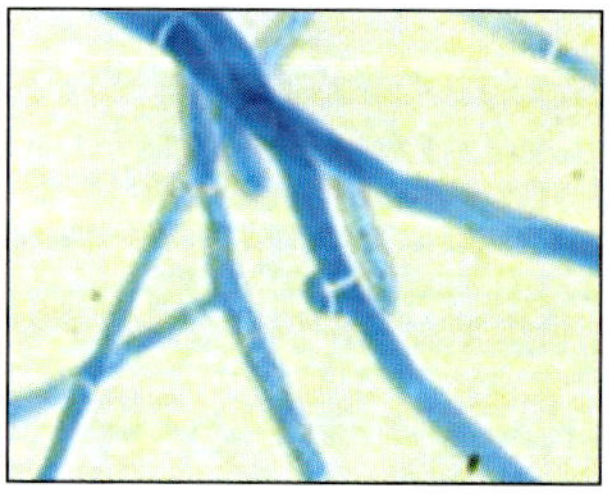

Clavate
Club shaped.

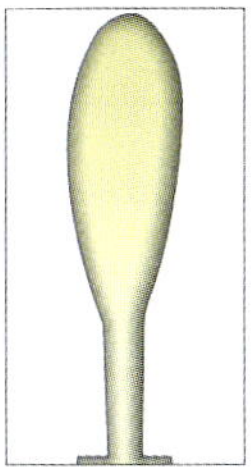

Cleistothecium
An enclosed fruiting body that contains randomly dispersed asci.

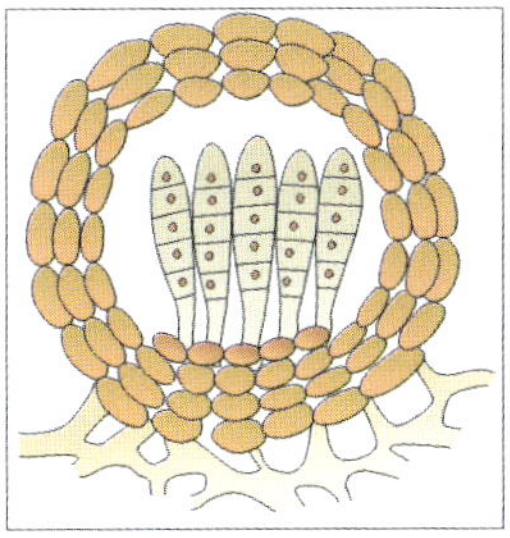

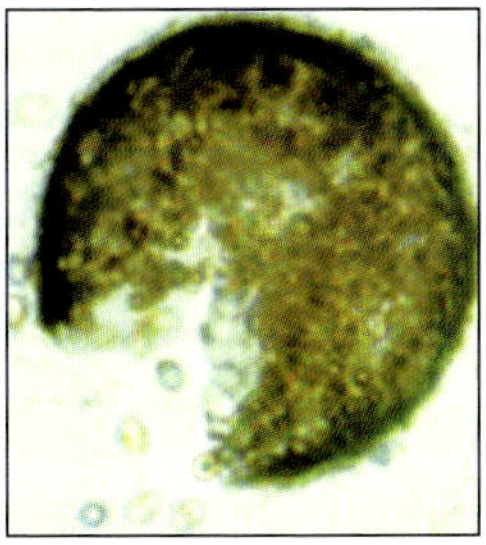

Coenocytic
Infrequently septate, multinucleate hyphae as in the zygomycetes.

Collarette
Cup-or funnel-shaped structure at the apex of a phialide, through which the conidia are produced.

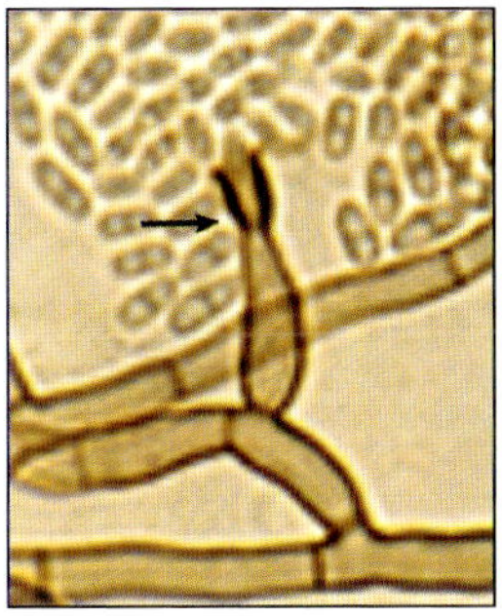

Columella (pl. columellae)
A sterile dome-like expansion at the apex of a sporangiophore.

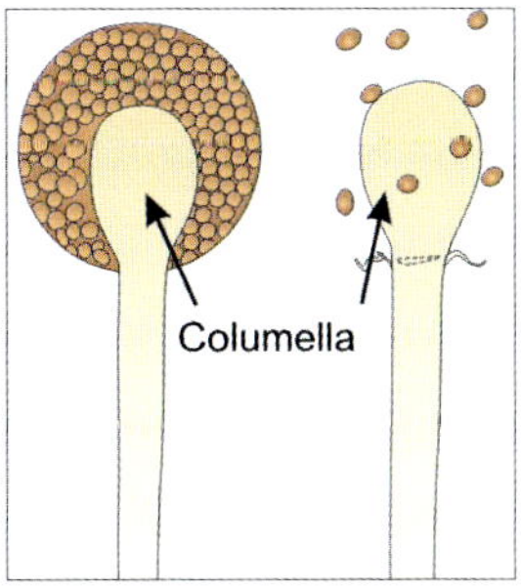

Conical
A sterile dome-like expansion at the apex of a sporangiophore.

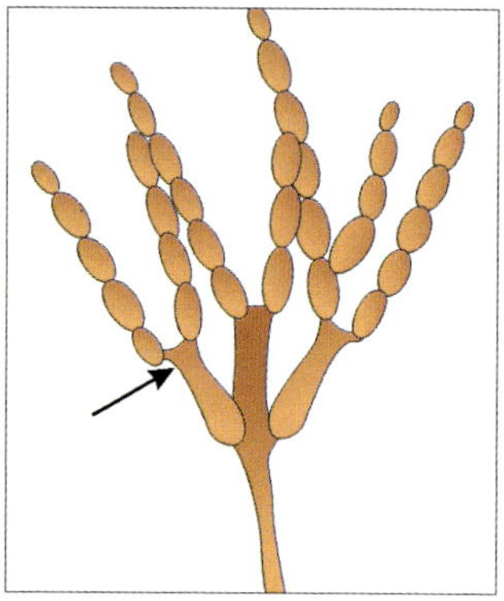

Conidiogenous cells
A cell that gives rise to conidia.

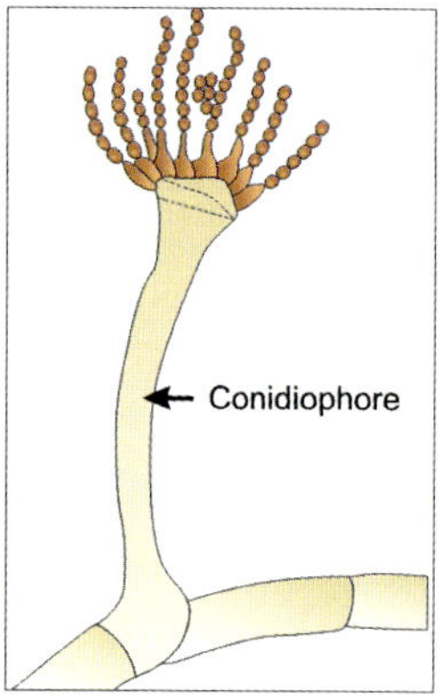

Conidiophore
Specialized, differentiated hyphal structure bearing conidia.

Conidium (pl. conidia)
Asexual propagule in Asco- or Basidiomycota produced on or in hypha or specialized supporting structure. It is not formed by cytoplasmic cleave, free-cell formation, or by conjugation.

Cottony
Loose, fragile aerial mycelium upto 5 mm high.

D

Denticle
A narrow delicate tooth- like conidium - bearing projection or peg.

Dematiaceous
Having brown to black conidia or hyphae.

Dimorphic
Displaying two morphological forms, one saprophytic and one parasitic.

Disjunctor cell
An empty cell between conidia that fragments/ undergoes lysis to promote the disarticulation of the conidia.

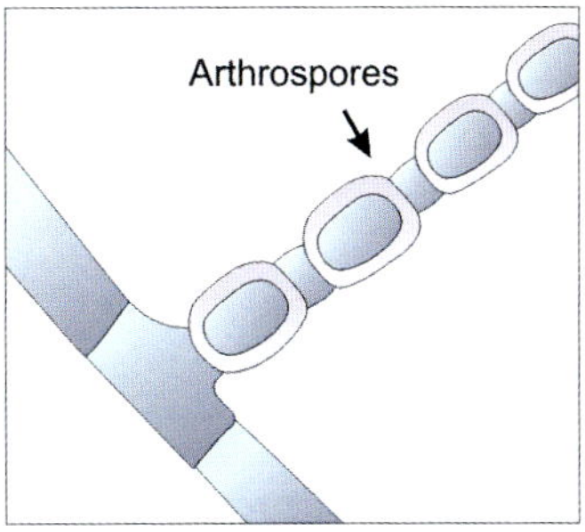

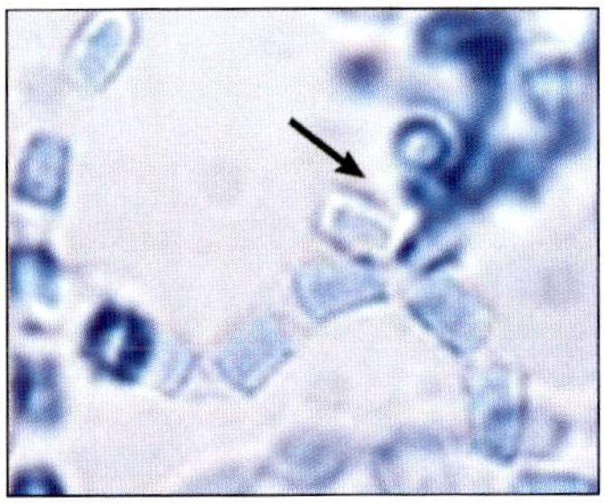

Distosepta
Conidia subdivided by inner wall layer only.

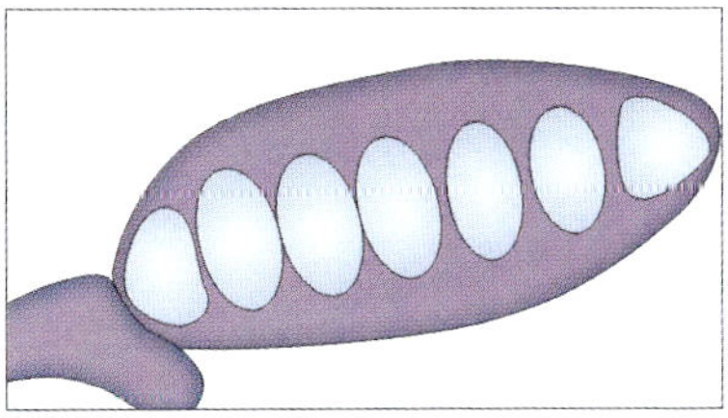

E

Echinulate
Covered with delicate spines

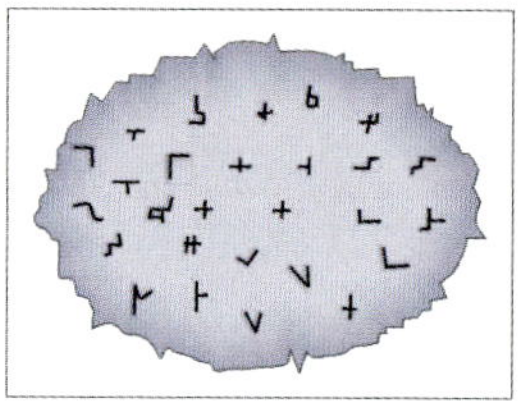

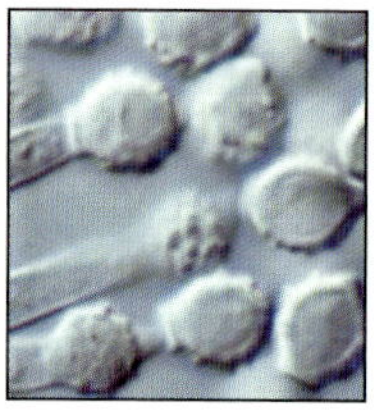

Endospore
A spore formed within a spherule by a cleavage process following karyogamy and mitosis.

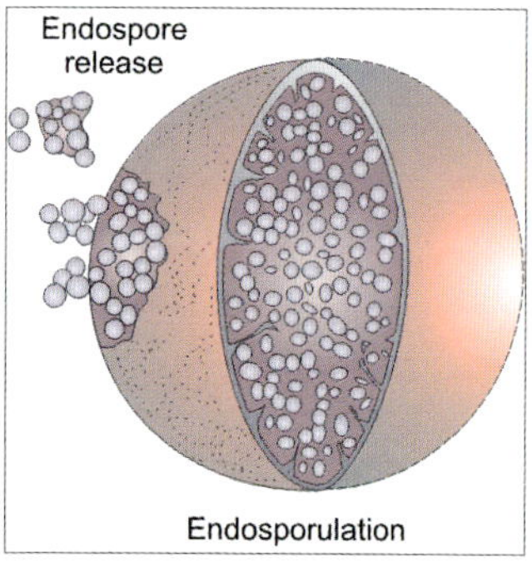

Exudate
Droplets of fluid formed on the surface of a colony.

F

Favic chandelier
A repeatedly branched cluster of hyphal apices that resembles a chandelier.

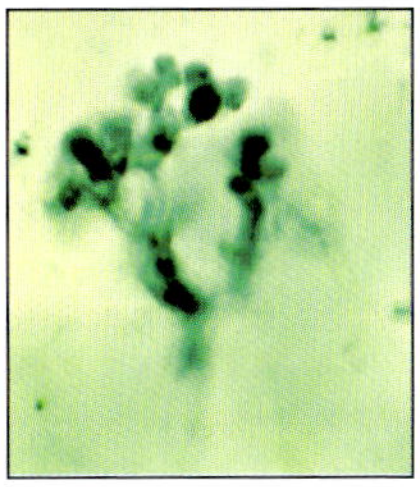

Fission
A discrete cell is divided with one or more septa, each segment becoming liberated as a separate cell.

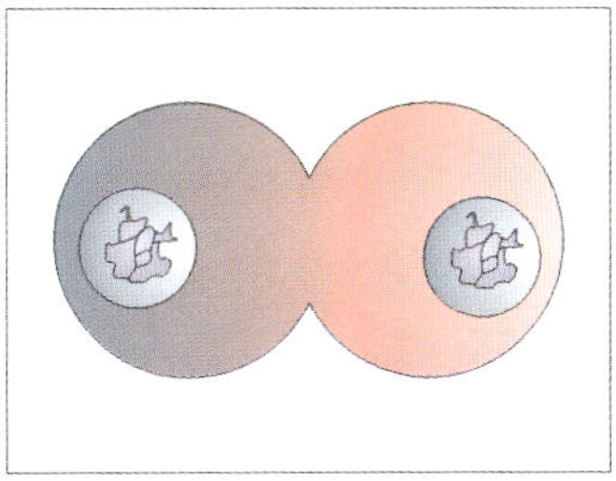

Fission arthroconidium
An arthroconidium that is released by fission through a double septum, eg: in *Geotrichum*.

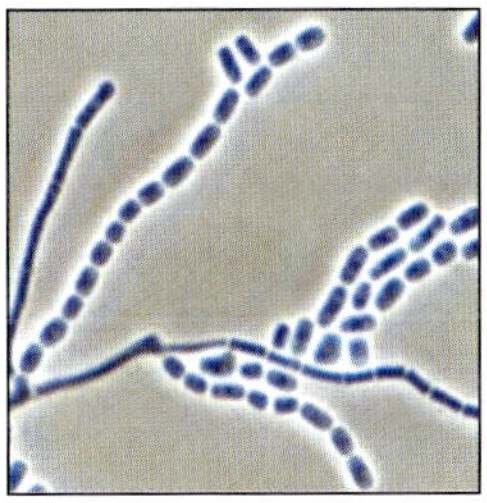

Flexuose
With smooth bends

Floccose
Having a cottony texture.

Foot cell
The base of a macrophialoconidium produced by a species of *Fusarium* having a heel-like projection; the base of the conidiophore of *Aspergillus* species where it merges with the hypha and resembles the heel and toes of a foot.

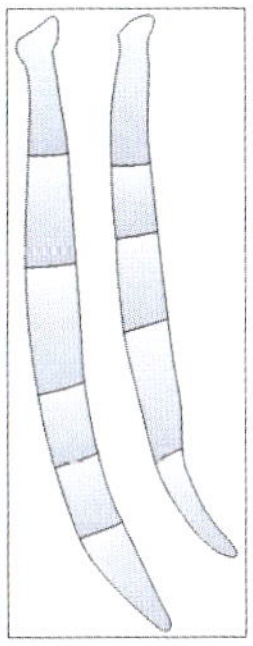

Fragmentation
Separation of a hyphae into conidia.

Fungus (pl. fungi)
A eukaryotic, unicellular to filamentous, achlorophyllous organism having an absorptive nutrition. A fungus reproduces by sexual, asexual, or both means.

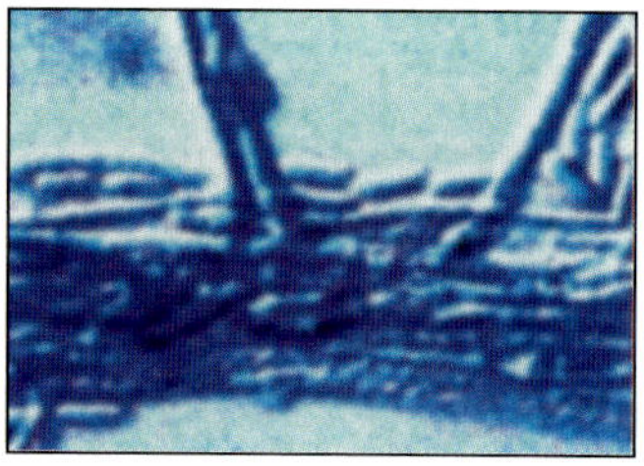

Funiculose
Aggregated into ropelike strands.

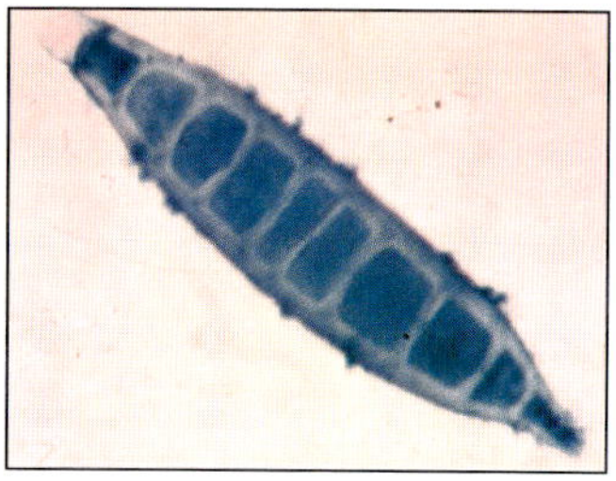

Fusiform
Spindle-shaped, swollen near the middle, strongly narrowed towards both ends.

G

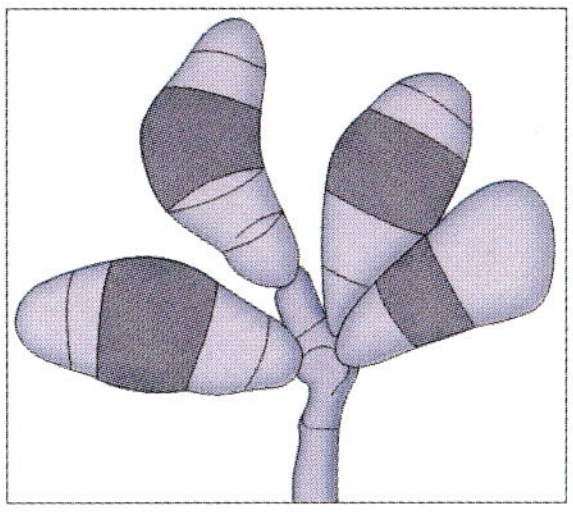

Geniculate
With repeated knee-like bents.

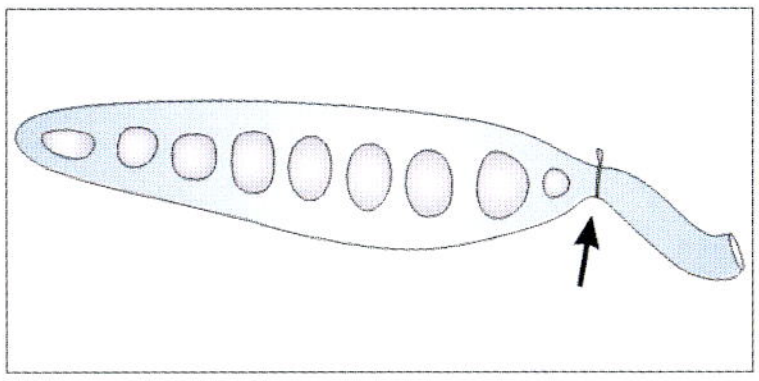

Germ pore
Circular thin-walled part of a propagule through which germination takes place.

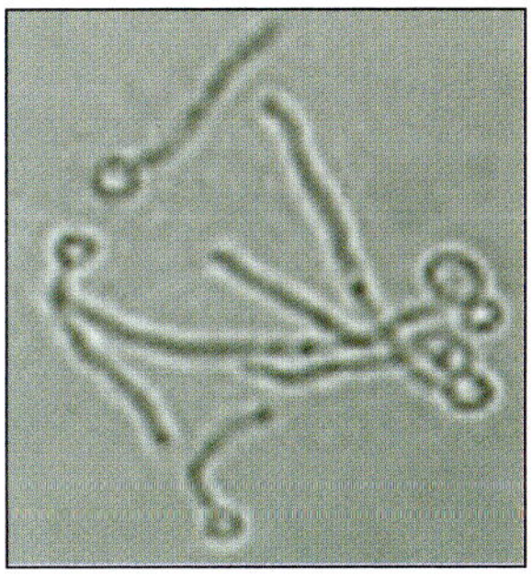

Germ tube
A hypha initially developing from a conidium or spore.

Glabrous
Smooth; (of colony), without aerial mycelium

H

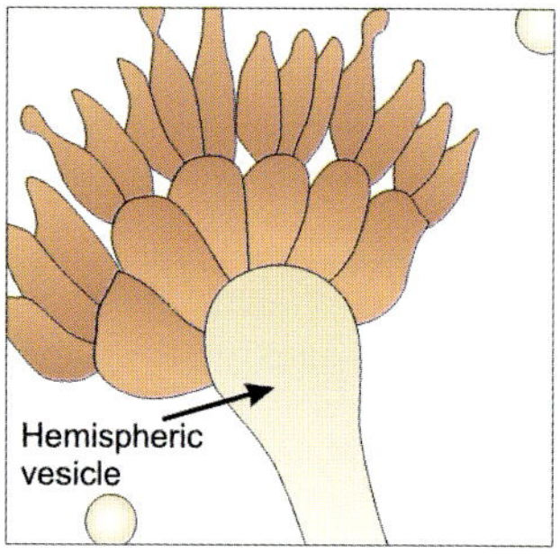

Hemispheric
Half of a sphere.

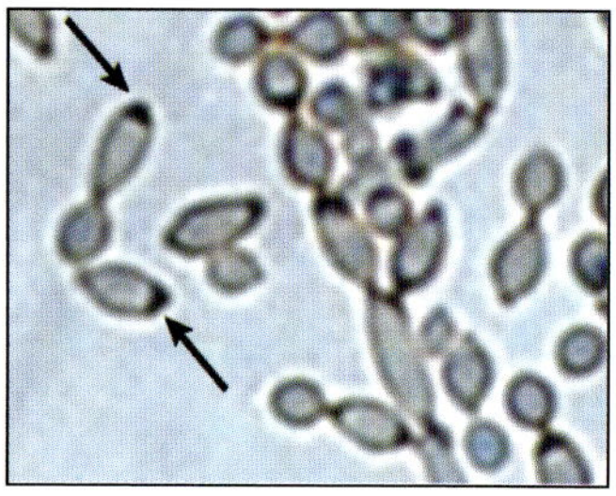

Hilum
Slightly prominent basal scar.

Homothallic
A fungus capable of sexual reproduction on a single thallus.

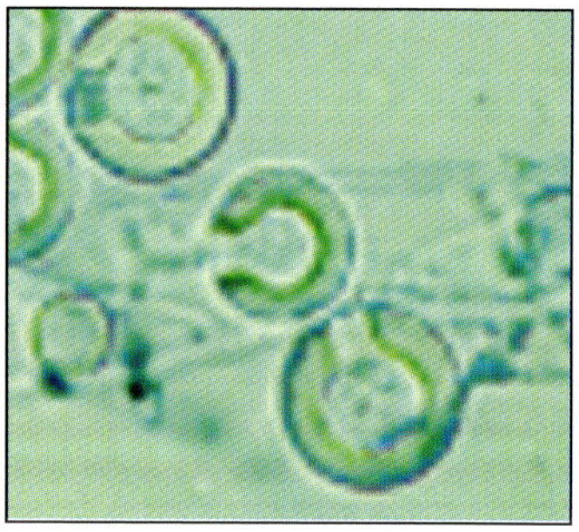

Hulle cells
Thick walled cells with characteristic thin walled pores,usually associated with cleistothecia of some species of *Aspergillus*.

Hyaline
Colorless, transparent.

Hypha
An individual filament of a fungus.

I

Intercalary
Incorporated in a mycelial filament, in between hyphal cells.

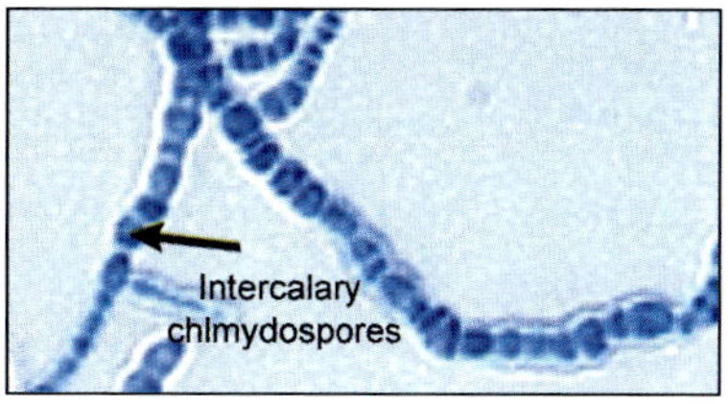

Internode
That portion of a hypha that is between two nodes.

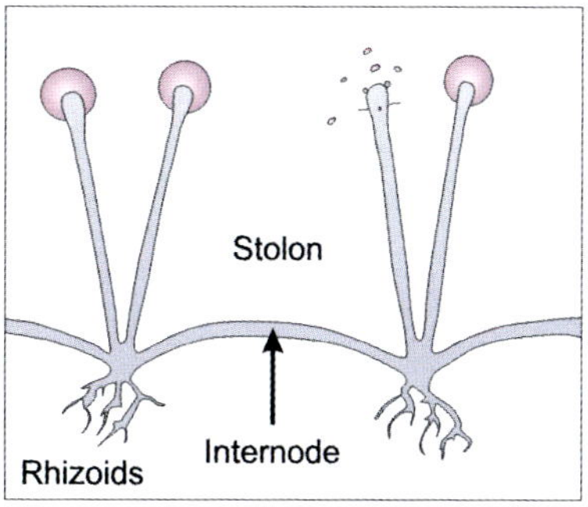

K

Karyogamy
Fusion of two nuclei during a sexual process.

L

Lanose
Wooly, with abundant loose, regular aerial mycelium.

Lenticular
Lens-shaped, circular in face view and ellipsoidal in lateral view.

Limoniform
Lemon-shaped, with small protrusions at the poles.

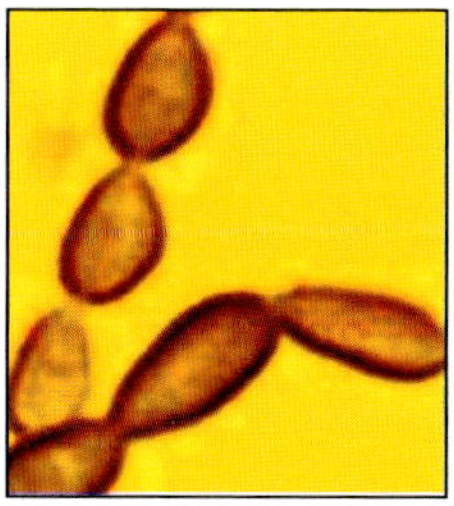

Lysis
Dissolution.

M

Macroconidium
The larger of two conidia of two different sizes that are produced in the same manner by a single fungus.

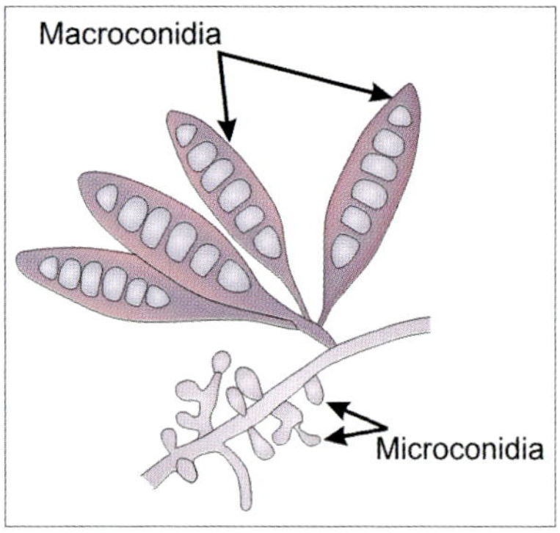

Merosporangium
A sporangium having its sporangiospores in a single row.

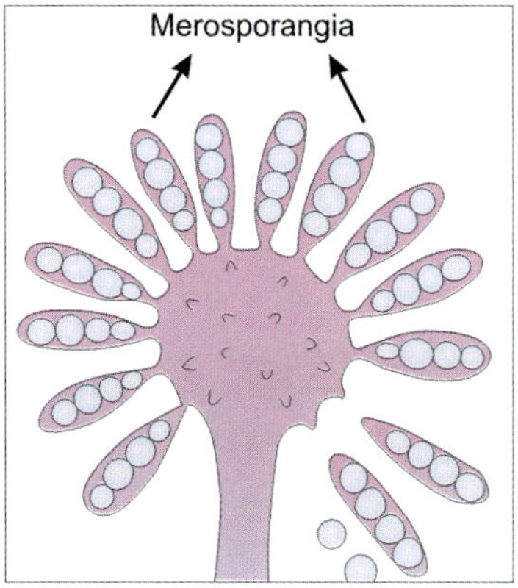

Metula
A sterile branch upon which phialides of some species of Aspergillus and Penicillium develop.

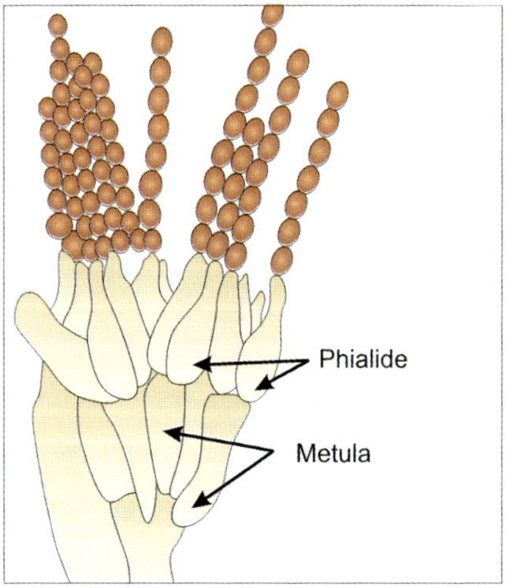

Microconidia
The smaller of two conidia of two different sizes that are produced in the same manner by a single fungus.

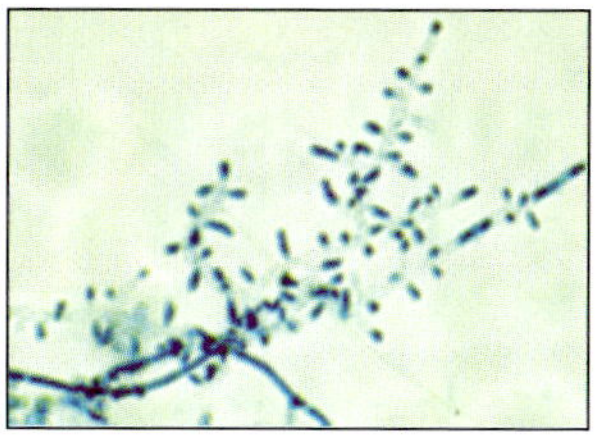

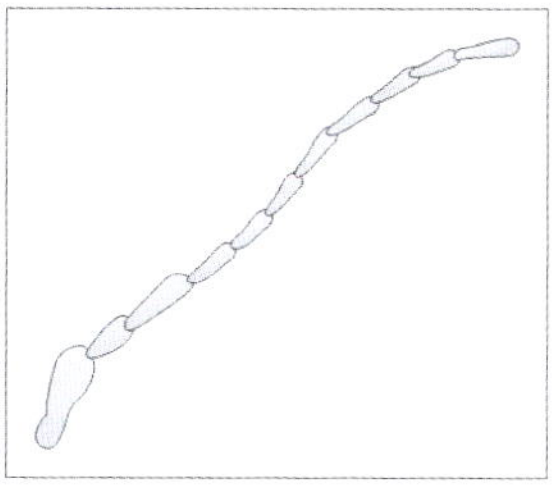

Moniliform
Coherent chain of cells.

Mould
A filamentous fungus.

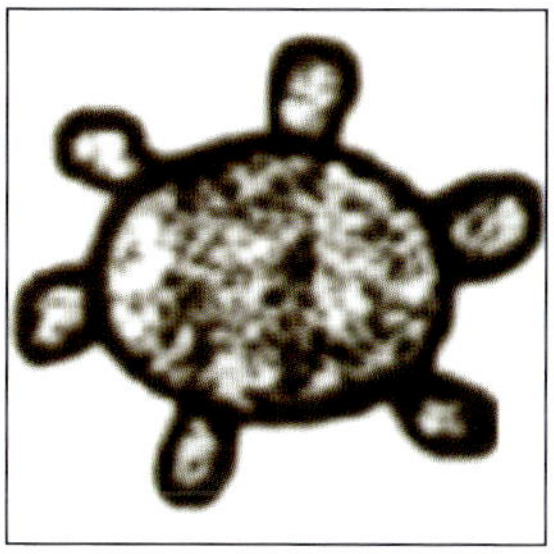

Multiple budding
Blastoconidia developing at different sites on the surface of a parent cell

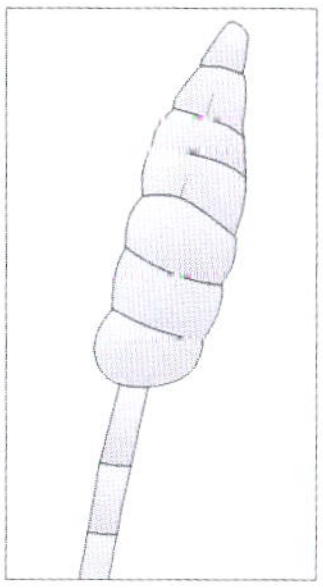

Muriform
Having vertical and horizontal septa.

Mycelium
The aggregated mass of hyphae making up a fungus.

Mycology
The branch of biology that deals with the study of fungi.

N

Node
Where a stolon touches a surface.

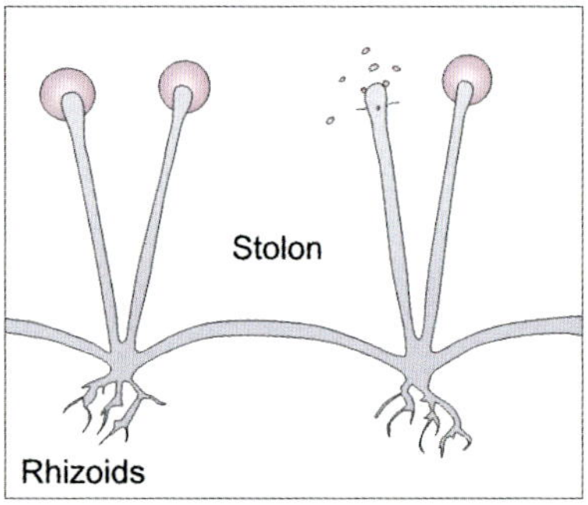

Nodular organ
A knot of hyphae that is often produced by dermatophytes.

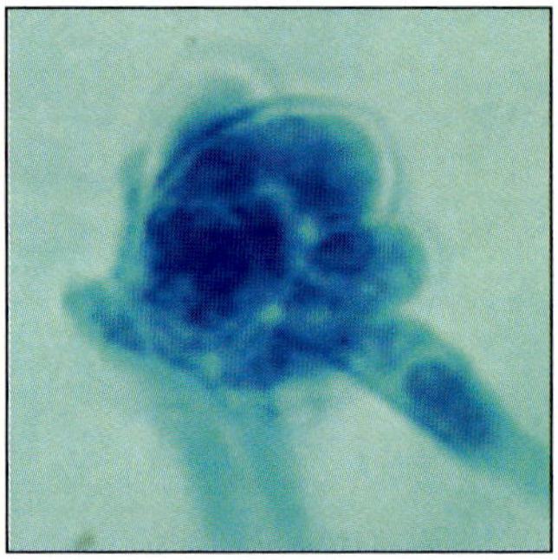

O

Obclavate
Club shaped in reverse.

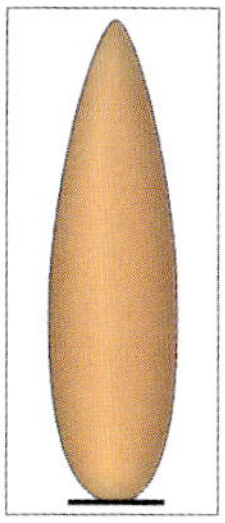

Obovoid
Egg shaped in reverse.

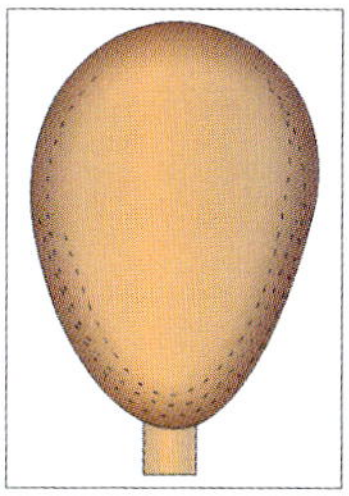

Olivaceous
Olive-grey in colour

Ostiole
An opening or pore in an ascocarp or a pycnidium.
See Perithecium

See perithecium

Oval
Egg shaped

P

Papilla (pl. papillae)
A small nipple-shaped elevation.

Penicillus:
The brush like conidiophore of *Penicillium*

Percurrent
Conidiogenous cell growth where a new axis grows through the previous apex.

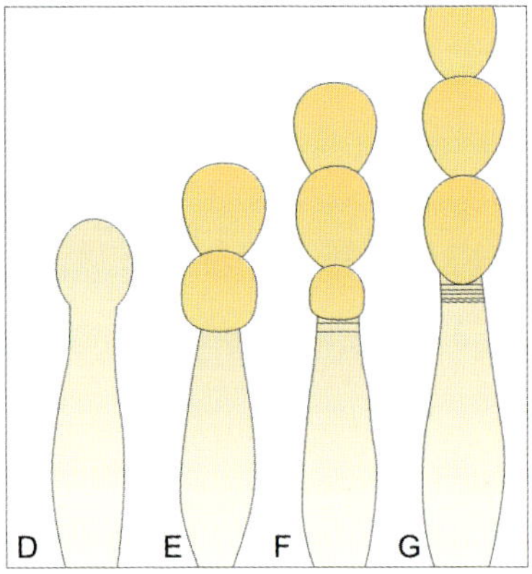

Perithecium
A fruiting body having asci in a basal group or as a layer; perithecia are usually flask shaped, with an opening through which the asci or ascospore escape.

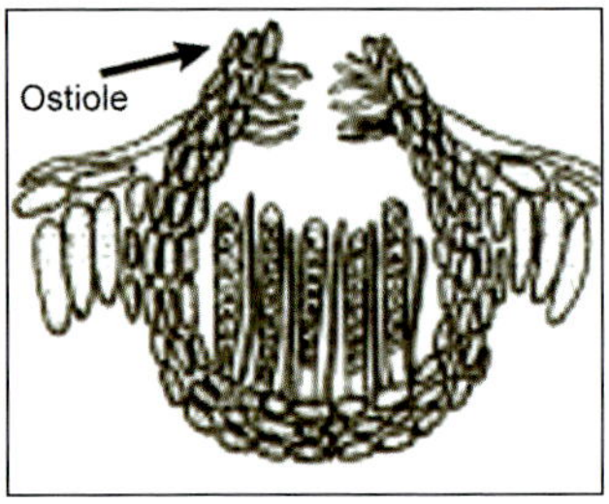

Phialide
A type of conidiogenous cell that gives rise to successive conidia from a fixed site in a basipetal manner. A phialide does not increase in length as the conidia are formed, and its apex does not become smaller in diameter. A collarette is often present at the apex of the phialide.

Phialoconidium
Propagule produced from a phialides.

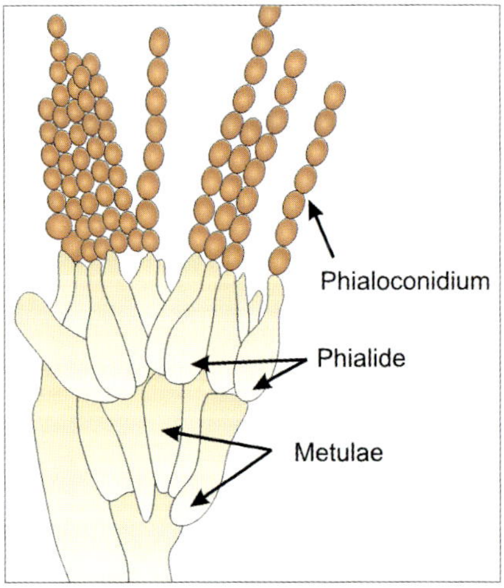

Pleomorphic
Having several forms. The term is also applied to dermatophyte colonies that become irreversibly sterile.

Polymorphic
Having several forms.

Pseudohypha
A series of blastoconidia that have remained attached to each other forming a filament. The blastoconidia are often elongated with the points of attachment between adjacent cells being constricted.

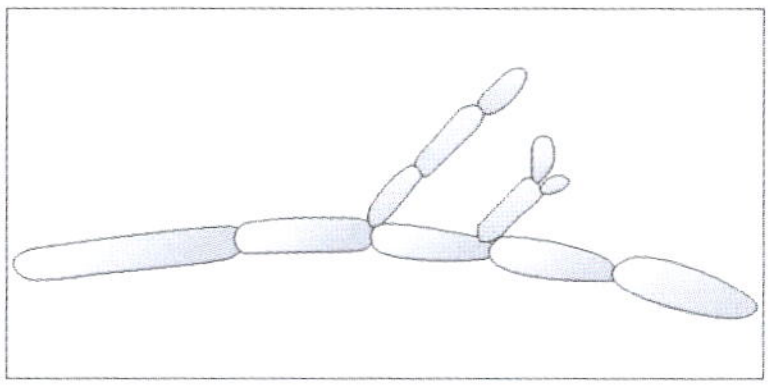

Pseudomycelium
A large amount of pseudohyphae.

Pycnidium
A sac-like fruiting body that gives rise to conidia within its central area.

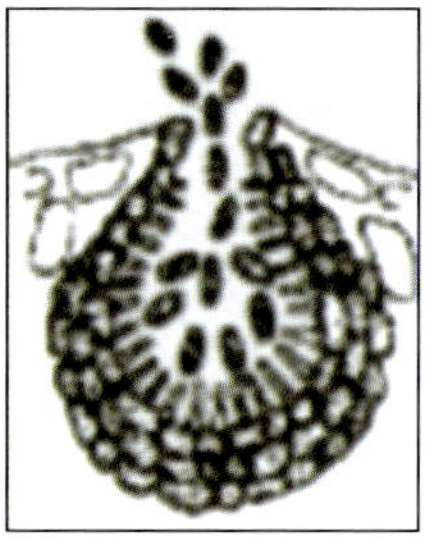

Pyriform
Pear shaped with narrow end down.

R

Rachis
An extension of a conidiogenous cell-bearing conidia.

Radiating
Spreading from a common center.

Rhizoid
Root-like structure with which the organism grows into the substrate.

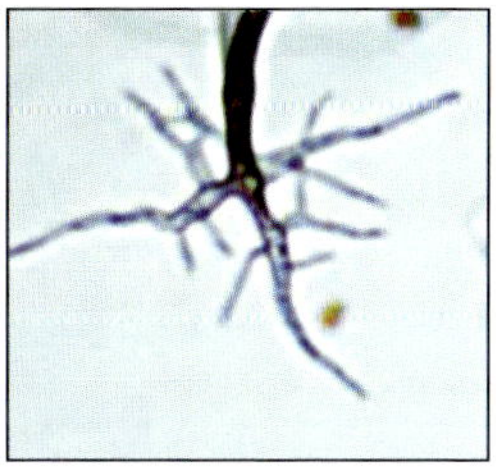

S

Sclerotia
An organized mass of hyphae that remains dormant during unfavorable conditions.

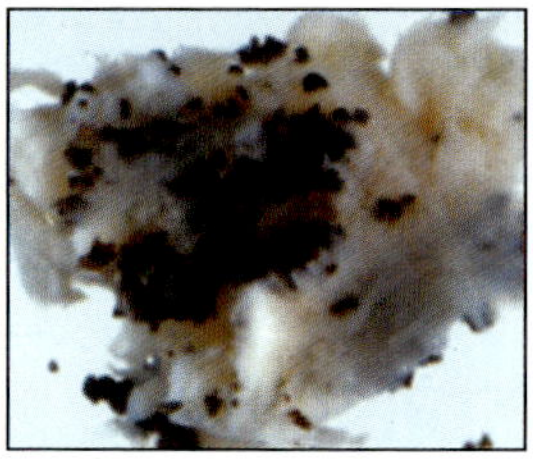

Sclerotia from a case of mycetoma

Seta (pl. setae)
A bristle or bristle-like structure.

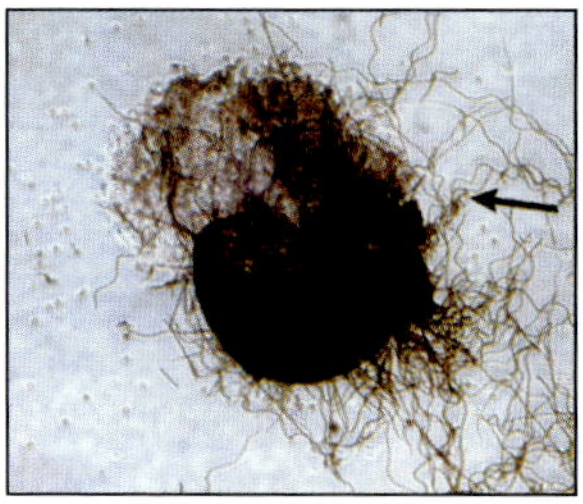

Shield cell
A conidium having the shape of a shield. Shield cells are commonly produced by members of the genus *Cladosporium*.

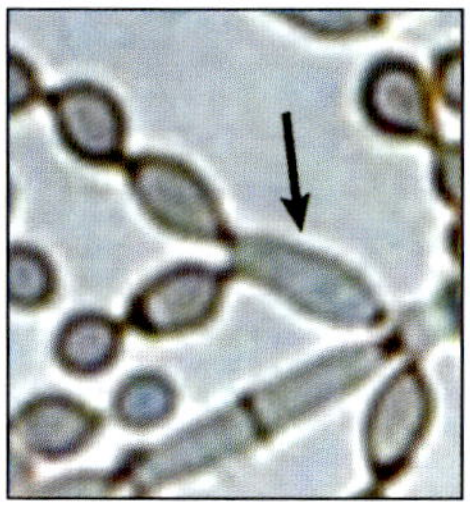

Solitary
Alone, only a single conidium being formed per conidiogenous cell.

Sporangiolum (pl. sporangiola)
A sporangium that contains a small number of sporangiospores. Some sporangiola may contain only one sporangiospore.

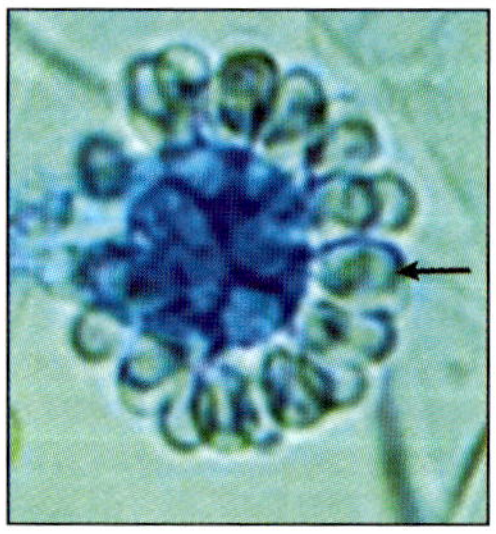

Sporangiophore
A specialized hypha that gives rise to a sporangium.

Sporangiospore
A spore that is formed by a cleavage process following karyogamy and mitosis in a sporangium.

Sporangium(pl. sporangia)
An asexual sac-like cell that has its entire content cleaved into sporangiospores.

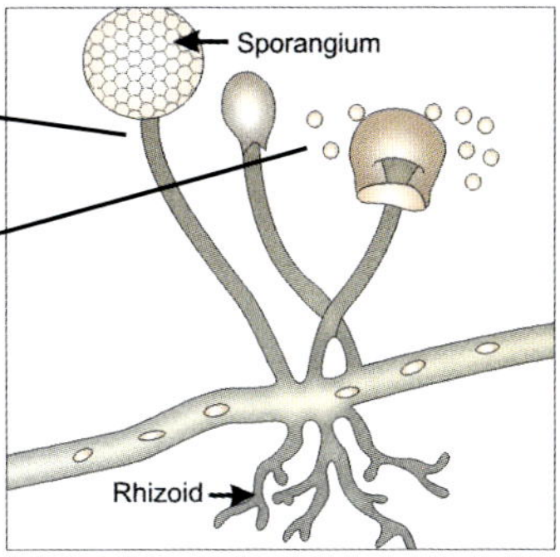

Spore
General term for a reproductive propagule in fungi; in higher fungi it is meiotic (in contrast to conidium)

Sporodochium (pl. sporodochia)
A cushion-like mat of hyphae bearing conidiophores over its surface, e.g. in *epicoccum*

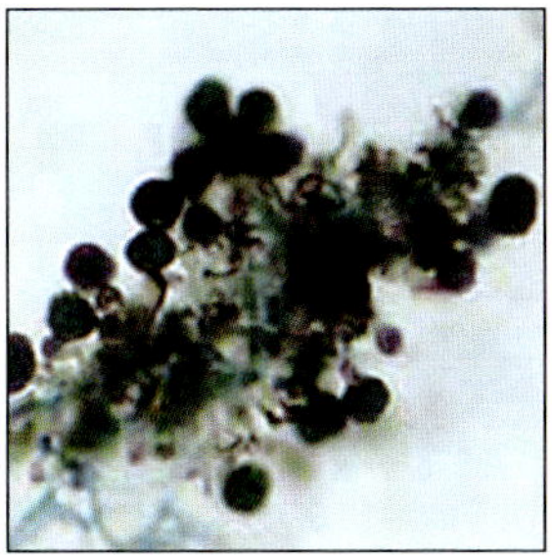

Sterigma
Slender, spine-like outgrowth of cell bearing a conidium.

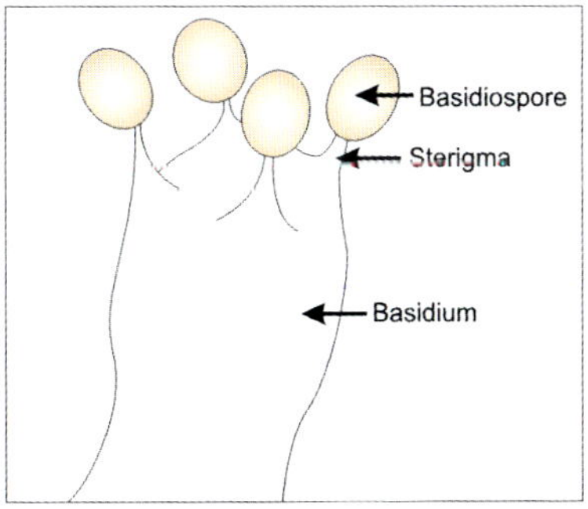

Stipe
Conidiophore bearing vesicle in *Aspergillus*.

Stolon
Horizontal hyphae growing along the surface of growth medium, a runner.

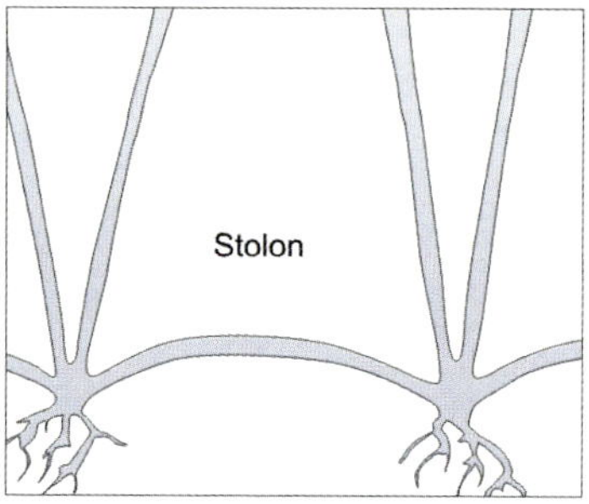

Subglobose
Almost round.

Submerge
Below the surface of the growth medium.

Sympodial
Pertaining to the growth of a conidiophore in which new successive lateral, subterminal apices of growth occur following successive conidium formation. Sympodial conidiophores are typically geniculate in appearance.

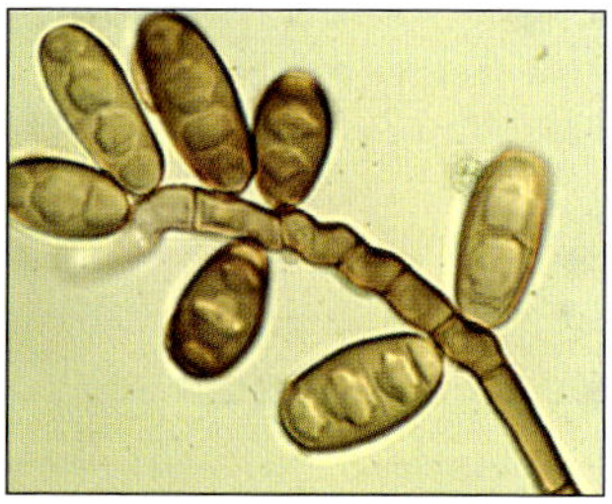

Synanamorph
Two or more distinct anatomic forms (anamorphs) produced by one fungus.

Synnema (pl. synnemata)
An erect macroscopic structure consisting of united conidiophores that bear conidia terminally, laterally, or in both ways.

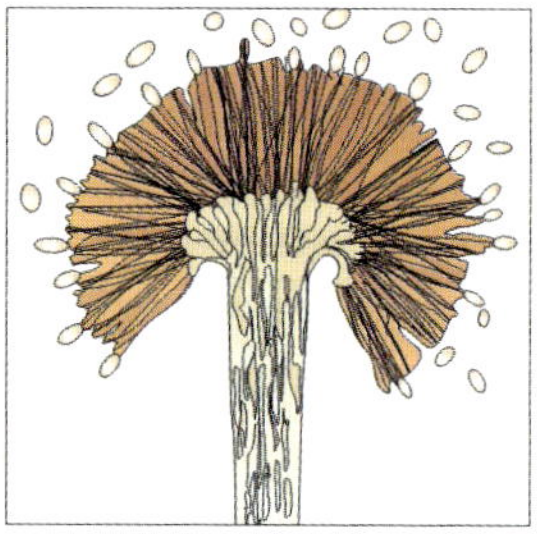

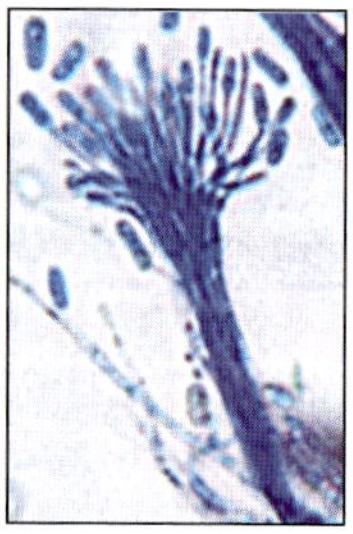

T

Teleomorph
A form based on a sexual state.

Truncate
With flat base, the scar being nearly as wide as the conidium.

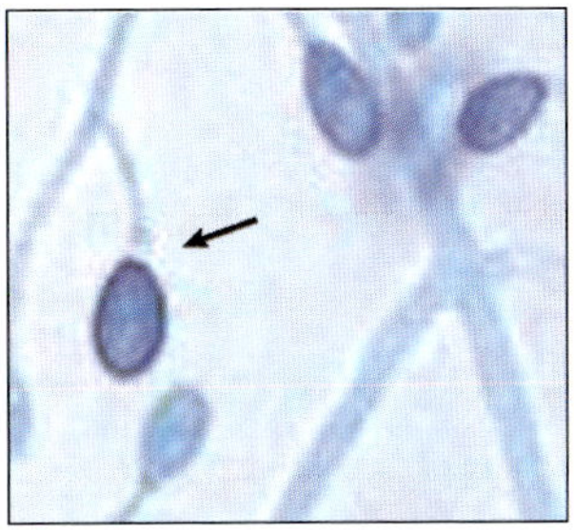

Tubercuate
Having finger-like or wart-like projections.

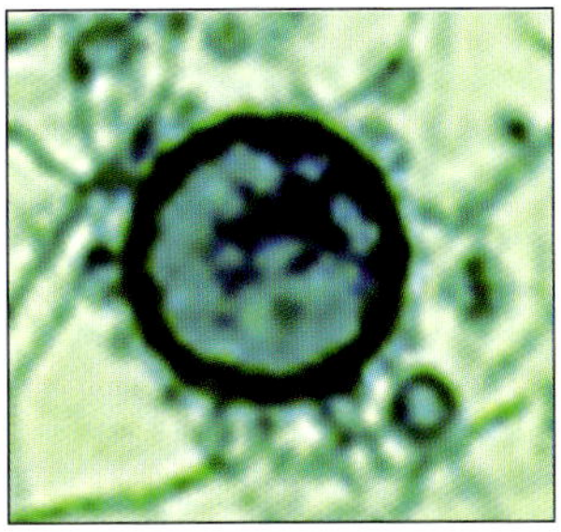

U

Unipolar budding
The development of conidia at one end of the parent cell.

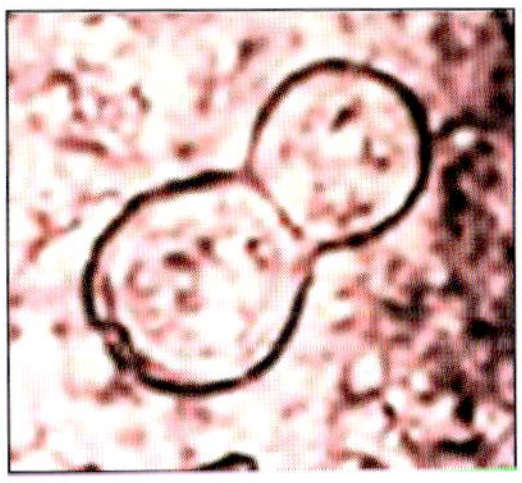

Uni seriate
In Aspergillus, single layer of phialides on vesicle; of ascospores within an ascus: in a single row.

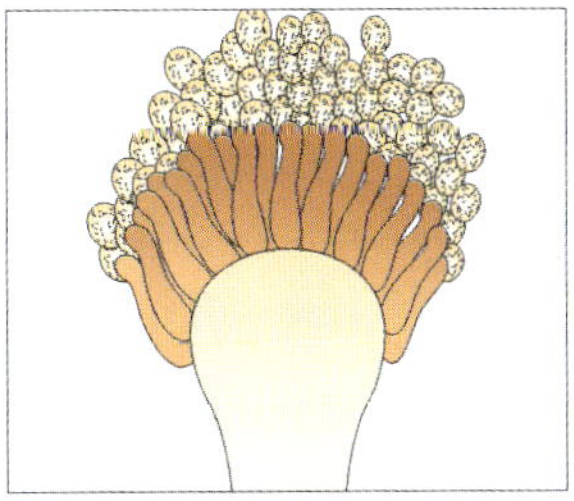

V

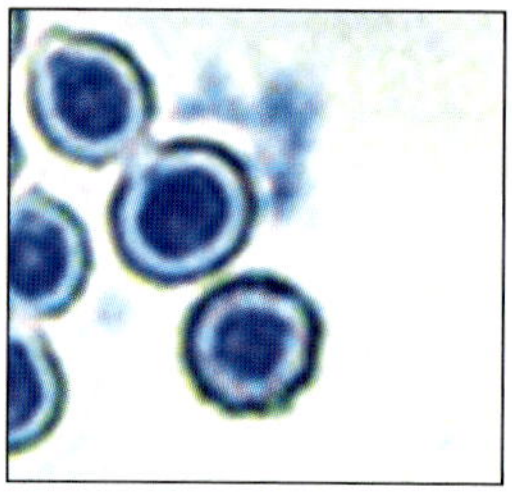

Verrucose
Distinctly and regularly rough-walled.

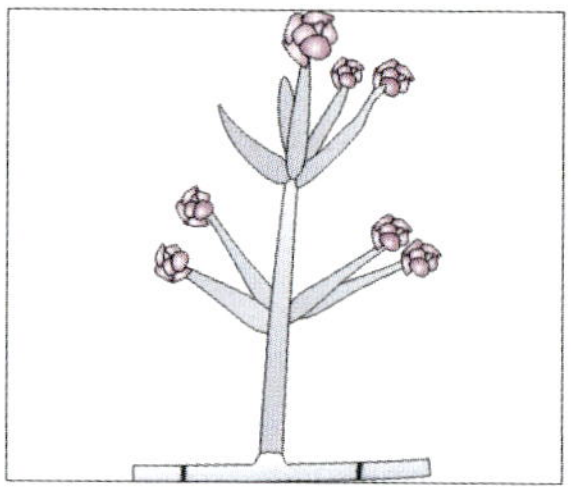

Verticil
A whorl of conidiogenous cells or conidiophores arising from a common point.

Verticillate
Having verticils.

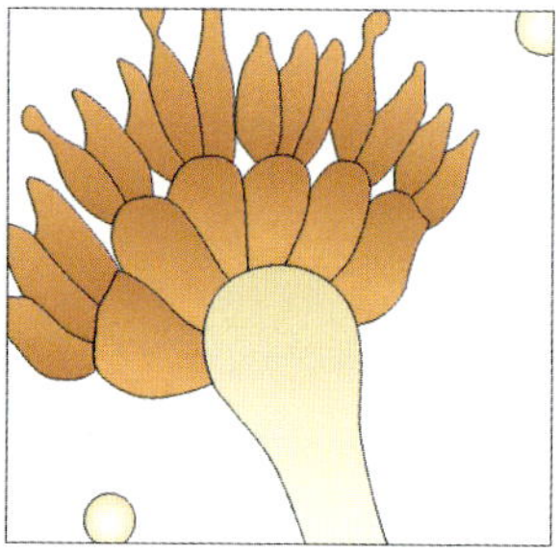

Vesicle
A swollen cell; the swollen apices of some conidiophores or sporangiophores.

Villose
Bearing long, hair-like appendages.

Y

Yeast
Unicellular budding fungus that reproduces by sexual, asexual or both means; mostly belonging to the Hemiascomycetes, but also to the Basidiomycota and occasionally to the filamentous Ascomycota ('black yeasts').

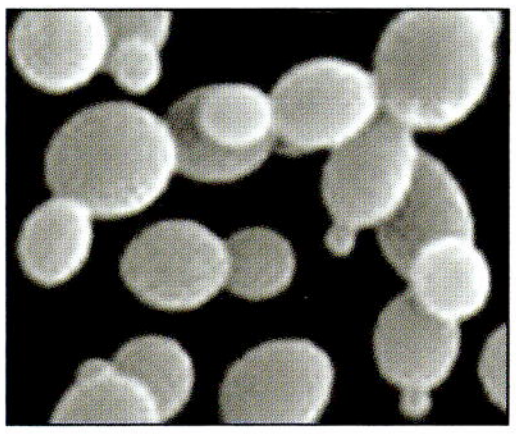

Yeast like
Pertaining to a unicellular budding fungus that reproduces by asexual means only

Z

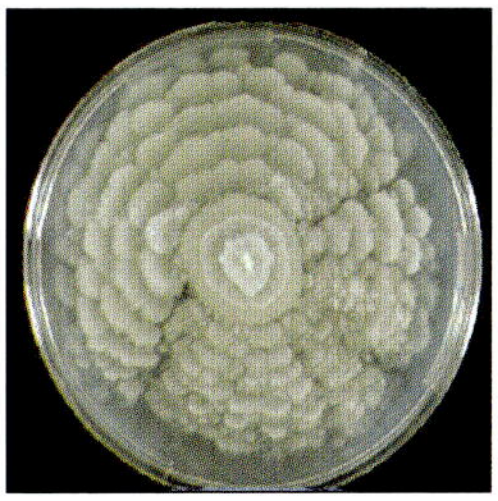

Zonate
Having concentric bands of color or growth.

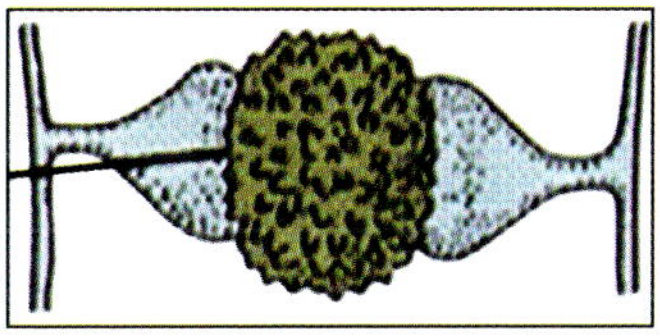

Zygospore
Resting spore resulting from the conjugation of hyphal tips in Zygomycota, in which karyogamy and meiosis takes place.

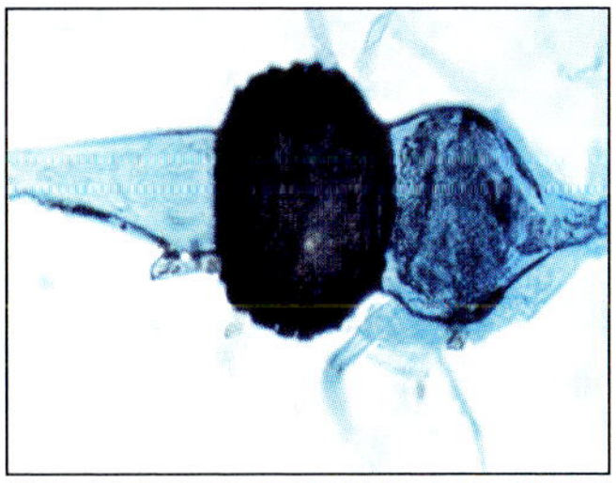

Index